# RAISING
# SUPERMAN!

# RAISING SUPERMAN!

*A Parent's Guide To Super-Special Children*

## AUTISM 101

*Real Life Secrets, Shortcuts, and "Cheat Codes"*
*Needed to Win the War against Autism!*

## HOWARD L. RODGERS

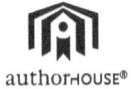

authorHOUSE®

*AuthorHouse*™
*1663 Liberty Drive*
*Bloomington, IN 47403*
*www.authorhouse.com*
*Phone: 1-800-839-8640*

*First published by AuthorHouse 3/1/2010*

*ISBN: 978-1-4490-8491-2 (e)*
*ISBN: 978-1-4490-8489-9 (sc)*
*ISBN: 978-1-4490-8490-5 (hc)*

*Library of Congress Control Number: 2010901952*

*Printed in the United States of America*
*Bloomington, Indiana*

*This book is printed on acid-free paper.*

# DEDICATION

This book is dedicated to Debbie, my wife. It is through her love, spirit, and dedication that all good things have come to pass in my life. This is also dedicated to Norman, my father and my son. Both have guided my life and shown me what's really important. Finally, this is for everyone who struggles with life's complex and sometimes unforgiving issues.

Here is a small drop of medicine created for those families faced with some of the worst that life can dish out. It's for all those folks struggling each and every day to improve their lives and the lives of those around them. Remember, it's only when you bump a coffee cup that you see what's really underneath the foam. So hold on tight!

*Here's to those who continue to struggle in the midst of severe adversity, hoping someday for just one of their prayers to be answered.*

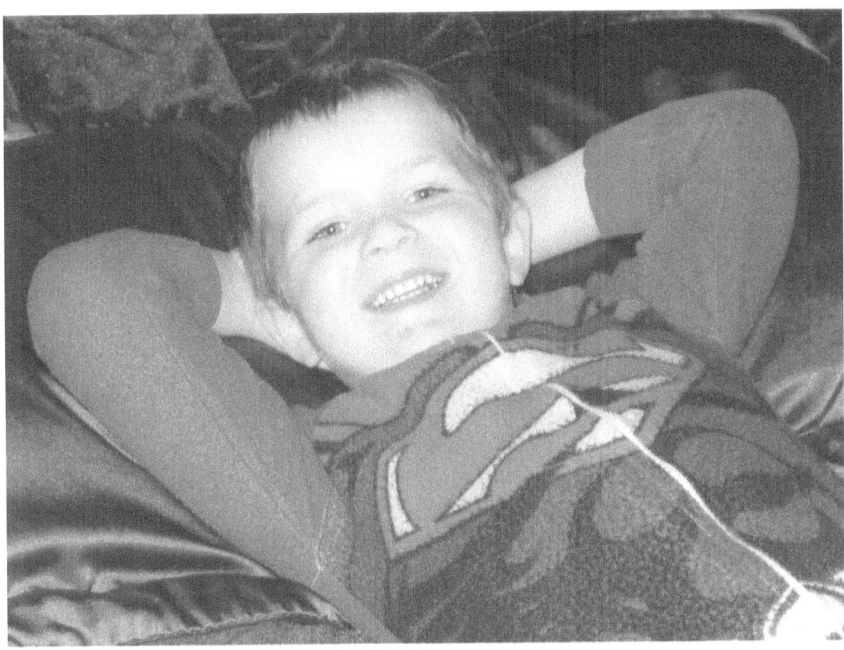

# CONTENTS

# Introduction

I want to ensure that everyone who picks up this book knows exactly what this book is about, and what it's not about. *Raising Superman!* is my attempt to share the lessons, blessings, and struggles that my family has experienced over the last sixteen years while raising our severely disabled, mentally retarded, and heavily autistic son.

It is not a book about positive thinking, hopeful outcomes, or magic wish-lists. It is a short, concise guide sharing many of the most important things we've either learned or realized as we worked through our struggles against autism, sometimes falling upon these items by accident. This guide borrows a lot of material from some very smart people, as none of us are intelligent or lucky enough to come up with all of life's answers by ourselves.

This book is intended to be a very useful, step-by-step, easy-to-read handbook for anyone who is raising a disabled child, those folks who have someone close to them doing the same, or anyone else wanting to learn more about what the families of severely disabled children are faced with.

It is not intended to provide medical advice, nor does it contain medical facts. In fact, most of this material is highly subjective and offers just an opinion. Over the years, we've found that most of what we've experienced as a family in raising our child has nothing to do with medical treatments. Remember, disabled children with cognitive and sensory impairments need very different kinds of love, attention, and care. So it's not surprising that successfully raising these children requires a different type of approach, if the family is to survive and flourish.

I originally was going to call this book *But What about the Rest of Us?* to focus on the fact that many people really struggle for a long time to find the right way to care for their severely disabled child. Although some disabled, autistic, or mentally retarded children have miraculous recoveries, the reality is that more often than not, most children with serious disabilities do not recover overnight. Families struggle for years trying to find the right mix of emotions, decisions, technologies, and supports to help safely raise and care for their child.

*The material in this book is* not *sugar-coated.* My only promise is that what you read in this book is the straight deal, as we lived it. Even when improvements are seen in a disabled child, it often takes years of focused, dedicated effort. So I wanted to share our lessons learned that deal with the issue of tackling life head on, as it falls out of the sky—in its raw form.

So what about the rest of us? The "rest of us" refers to those of us who want to do the very best for our disabled children but are faced with a very difficult set of circumstances, problems, and emotions when things don't magically get better overnight. This book is about keeping your sanity in a very insane situation, when even doctors, medicines, prayers, and tears don't help.

Successfully raising any child is difficult, at best. However, successfully raising a severely autistic child can be emotionally, spiritually, and financially draining. For those who attempt to do this as a single parent, this guide will hopefully provide you with a shortcut to some items that should help. For those who struggle to do this as a partnership in marriage, this material should help you keep your marriage together and allow you to focus on what's really important. Finally, for those who read it and do not agree with the material, that's fine too. Having an opinion, even a contrary one, is vital to the success of raising a disabled child.

The statements you're about to read are my opinion as to what worked for us. Your personal experience will most likely be different. However, one thing is certain: raising a child with a disability takes time, focus, and energy. I'm writing this first book to provide some immediate shortcuts, tricks, and "cheat sheets" as to what worked best for our family. This is triage for one of life's major tragedies, developed to help others find their way on the roller coaster of life while immersed in the fog of autism.

If you find that just one item in this book helps you improve your life, your child, or your family, then my effort was totally successful. In my second book, *Ten-inch Nails*, I'll cover the graduate-level autism 401 challenge. The second book explores the deeper emotional, financial, and spiritual challenges that come with this war, including the painful experiences, incredible revelations, and tearful results as a resource to help those fighting their own personal autism battles.

I wish you the best on whatever life brings you and your family. Remember, we're all here for a reason. We just won't know the reason until we leave for our next tour of duty.

Meanwhile, enjoy the ride!

*Howard L. Rodgers*

# RAISING
# SUPERMAN!

# CHAPTER 1

# IT'S A BOY!

I still remember the day our first son was born, as it feels like it happened yesterday. My wife was lying on the operating table having an emergency C-section. Her eyes were focused sharply on mine—peering deep into my soul. You could feel the emotional electricity shooting throughout the room. Tears streamed down both our faces when the doctor finally looked over at us and said, "It's a boy."

All our hopes and dreams had come true in that one small instant of time. My head was instantly filled with all kinds of positive thoughts about how this small child would change the world. He was so tiny and precious. He was my son! It was the happiest moment of my life.

Then reality came back—for a very long visit.

Over the next few months, we began to experience the realization that something was terribly wrong, although we couldn't quite put our finger on what it was. We weren't sure what was happening, as this was our first child, so we had nothing to compare these events to. Our son had a high fever just after receiving some shots. He cried (and cried and cried), and all our doctors told us was "You're new parents and this is normal. Just walk with him." So we did. I recall being up for weeks at a time, walking up and down the hallway, probably covering twenty miles of distance in one week. Despite all our effort, nothing helped.

Finally my son began crawling, but not consistently. He also began speaking but quickly lost this ability. Over the next two years, we sought the help of a variety of specialists. This finally resulted in us being told, "Your child has severe autism and mental retardation." It was not just any form of autism. He had very severe autism with many sensory and cognitive problems.

We didn't even know what this meant, but we knew it wasn't good. In fact, per the feedback we heard, our son had the worst case of autism the doctors and specialists at Johns Hopkins had ever seen. He was violent and often very mean. We had to wear a face shield to play with him, as he'd try to hurt us when we got near him. This wasn't the child I had hoped and dreamed for. It was some kind of nightmare I couldn't even deal with. And it didn't appear there was anything we could do to help him recover, despite reaching out for as many medical opinions and treatments as possible.

The day we realized what "having autism" meant was one of the worst days of my life. I remember crying and worrying and crying some more. All the hopes and dreams we had for our son went crashing down like a house of cards, and what we were left with was a child who needed more help than we could ever imagine. Despite many doctors and therapists telling us, "Don't worry, he'll improve," he didn't. None of them could ever imagine or describe the pain and anguish we were destined to face.

I want to stop here and say that things did actually improve—but it was a long, hard road to endure. Remember, I said in the introduction that I would tell this as it is, without sugar-coating it. I refuse to tell you, "It's not that bad," as believe me, it was that bad. However, there were a few things we did that really helped, and despite this child being really sick, we were determined to stick it out with him.

He needed our love and care, and we were determined to provide it to him, no matter what that meant. So I want to make sure that everyone reading this book realizes that from this point forward, we won't focus on the horrible, tormenting emotions that accompanied this event. We will focus on what really made things better—for him, for us, and for our family.

Medically, I think it's fair to say that only two things helped—and those were unapproved, unorthodox forms of treatment. I'll share what those were later in this book. Conventional medicine really had nothing to offer us. It's not that the doctors didn't try, as they tried very hard. Aside from some focused behavioral therapy (which took years and years to implement), nothing provided the quick fix or recovery we were hoping for. In fact, most of the medicines and treatments we tried either made our son worse or had no effect at all. So it seemed we were on our own, which was very scary to say the least.

So here we go. The following items are a quick guide to what worked for us. I'm keeping this brief and to the point, as I know a few things for sure. If you're a parent trying to raise a disabled child like we were doing, you don't have a lot of time to read useless material. Second, if you're a single parent trying to raise this type of child by yourself, your situation is even more challenging than what we went through. If this is the case, then I commend your dedication and love for your child. Last, if you're a family member trying to understand what someone else is going through, you also need to read the actual feedback to understand what we went through.

Remember, this is only our experience as to what worked for us. It's okay to disagree, take a contrary view, or decide that I'm wrong. Having an opinion as to how you want to raise your child is the first step in ensuring the results are what you want to see. Without an opinion, you'll be swayed by everyone who comes along and probably make the wrong choices. Finally, if you experience what we went through, you'll see that very few people on the planet at best have any idea what you're dealing with. So your opinion is probably more accurate than anyone else's opinion.

The key is to become a great advocate for your child. After all, they may be unable to speak or think for themselves. So it's up to you to get the right mix of items into a specialized environment for his or her safety and success. As we describe our experience, it will become clearer as to what being a great advocate for your child means, and what tasks it involves.

# CHAPTER 2

# DON'T DO
# THE BLAME GAME

The first realization came to me after years of struggling with what happened to our son. This may seem like a trivial matter, but it's not. At first, I didn't even realize I was carrying this around with me. However, it significantly prevented me from taking on some of the challenges we were faced with. I was blaming myself for what happened. Maybe not consciously, but definitely unconsciously there was a heaviness in my heart, and I felt somewhat responsible for what had occurred.

Depending on your specific circumstances, it's normal to feel like some part of what occurred is your fault. If you're the mother who carried a child, you may feel like you did something wrong during the pregnancy. If you're the father, you may feel like you did or didn't do something that contributed to the problem. Either way, these feelings are natural. However, it's critical that you put this past you immediately and get over it. Otherwise, it will continue to impact your ability to care for your child and may hinder future progress and improvement.

Our son came down with autism and mental retardation as a result of the shots he received (or so we think, as medically it's impossible to prove). Regardless of what others said, I felt as if I was responsible for him getting these shots. I carried this guilt with me for many, many years. Remember, I was the one who approved him getting the shots. I was the one who called the doctors and didn't push the issue hard enough regarding his fever, his crying, and his lack of recovery. I was the one who held him walking back and forth, all the while hoping things would improve. But things didn't improve. I felt as if I was the one who stuck the knife into my son's head—condemning him and our family to a life of torment, struggle, and anguish. And it *was* my fault, as I could have said no to the shots.

Many of you reading this may think, *Well this is just stupid. Of course it's not his fault, as no one could have possibly known what would occur.* As stupid as it sounds, I felt as if it was partly my fault, and inside I carried this guilt for years. I'm a professional with a technical degree, two masters degrees, and years of life experiences. None of these credentials could save me from the guilt and torment I carried when all this went down. Rationalizing the facts didn't help, as emotionally I had it in for myself. It was only through years of struggling that I came to the realization that you can't do the blame game or you further hurt your child. And here's why.

First, all things happen for a reason. It is very likely that my son may have developed this condition as a result of something other than the shots. No one knows for sure. Hind sight being 20/20, of course I think I should have stopped the shots from occurring. However, in the moment it occurred, I had him receive the shots so he could be protected from illness and disease. The intent was good—and no matter what the results were, we can only do our best with the information we have when given life's choices.

However, this is the real reason you can't do the blame game. No matter what I did or didn't do, blaming myself would not help improve the outcome. Whether or not I was responsible for what happened was irrelevant. What was relevant was that my son required significant help and needed for me to be at my best. Carrying the blame game around for years prevented me from making some of the good choices that would eventually help my son improve. It was a huge distraction preventing me from focusing on things that really mattered with respect to improving my son's condition. The blame clouded my thinking, emotionally drained me, and prevented my relationship with my son from fully developing until years later.

Consider this shortcut number one—*drop the blame game.* Whether it was your fault, the fault of your spouse, someone else's fault, or no one's fault at all, it really doesn't matter. Move on and focus on working with what you have in front of you. The decisions and actions you need to make require your full attention. You can't give your best to your child if you're walking around with a head full of guilt.

Remember, this is something *you* need to do, as no one else can make this happen. You need to really understand that for the best outcome of your child, you need to let go of the blame game, drop the guilt, forgive whoever needs to be forgiven, and move on. It's more difficult than it sounds, but this is absolutely vital for you to be at your very best when working to help your child. Otherwise, you'll always be half-heartedly engaging on the hard decisions that need to be made. You'll second guess every tough decision you make. You'll worry that round two of more bad decisions is just around the corner. And you will always be distracted from providing your full focus and attention on your child's needs. It'll prevent you from living your life. And worse, it'll prevent your child from getting the maximum care and love you need to provide.

So make this priority one, and realize that the only thing you should blame yourself for is not giving your child all the love and attention deserved from this point moving forward. After all, we can't change the past, and the future is uncertain. The present is the only thing we can directly impact, and it needs your focused attention right now.

# CHAPTER 3

# EXPECT TO BE DIFFERENT AS A PERSON, AS A PARENT, AND AS A FAMILY

This next step is something that many people have difficulty with, but whether you openly embrace it or not, it'll eventually happen. As the parent of a severely disabled or handicapped child, you need to recognize that your life and your actions will be very different from those around you. Things that tend to be simple decisions for other families may be extremely challenging or impossible for your family to do.

Let me begin by providing some examples, as this may help clarify what I'm referring to. Our son was very difficult to transport and next to impossible to control. As a result, some of our routine tasks (like shopping, visiting with family, etc.) became very difficult or impossible to engage in.

We eventually had to develop a routine where my wife went shopping while my son was at school or when I was home to supervise him. Why did we do this? It was the result of my wife being continuously bombarded by people telling her, "Please control your son." I can't tell you how many times she came home telling me about some store manager asking her to "take control of her son" or asking her, "Don't you discipline him?" At one point, we thought about printing up cards we could hand out saying, "Our son is disabled and whatever you think about his outbursts, you're wrong. So please mind your own business!" But in the end, it was just simpler to avoid the situation altogether.

Restructuring our shopping routine was one thing, but dealing with the family visits was another thing altogether. Once our son got to about seven years of age, he became very destructive and required continuous supervision with positive environmental controls. He also wasn't potty trained. When a child is two years old and not potty trained, it's a nuisance. When he's ten years old and not potty trained, it can be a major disaster. Each night, he would take the contents of his diaper and throw it all over his room, smear it all over himself, the floor, the walls, the ceiling, and … well, you get the picture. How do you describe this to your family members who are asking you, "So why don't you come down to visit for a while?"

We were faced with some very difficult decisions. Do we try to take this child outside of his tightly controlled environment, or adjust our lives so that we maintain him in the easiest, most effective/safe environment we could construct for him? We went with the second approach—keeping him (and ourselves) in our home environment, sacrificing the family visits.

This was very difficult, and to this day some of our family members probably do not understand. They may think that we think we are "too good to be with them." Or they may think we don't care about them. To be honest, I'm not sure what most of them think, aside from the fact that we're loners who don't visit them anymore. But none of them can even imagine the difficulty we face on a daily basis to just live with this child. Hopefully, they know we love them all dearly and appreciate all their help, support, and understanding as we've worked through these issues.

We had to make some very drastic adjustments in our life. For example, it became very obvious to us early in the game that we could not travel with our son—either on vacation or in any capacity. So we fixed up our home as our vacation spot. We put in a hot tub, sauna, tanning bed, pool, and other items to make our home much more enjoyable. To be honest, sometimes it still feels like we're tied to a prison, but at least it's a nice prison. Our home looks very different than our neighbor's homes, which ties to the theme of expect to be different. Outsiders probably see our home and think we're "toy crazy." But in fact, this is our attempt to not go crazy by having what we need, where we need it, when we need it.

We also had to modify the living conditions for our son, so we could easily address his "super-special messes." Eventually, we had his room covered floor to ceiling with one-inch plywood with Formica covering on top, so it's all like one big countertop. This was the only way we could easily clean up his messes and keep him from punching holes in the drywall. Remember, this chapter is about realizing you're going to be different. Different may mean adjusting your schedules so you don't aggravate behavioral issues by forcing your child into a public setting. Different may mean that you have commercial-sized cleaning equipment in your home to address the commercial-sized messes your child creates. Different may mean that your family vacation takes place outside in your fenced-in yard, as opposed to being at the beach or other public setting.

Each of these items revolves around choices, with the choices for your child coming first. So the meat and potatoes of this chapter are about just realizing you will be different—very different than those around you. So just get over it, move on, and do what you need to do to best care for your child, your family, and yourself. You can't worry about what other people think, or you and your child will suffer. Those who love you will understand, or maybe they won't. In the end, it really doesn't matter. What matters is that you and your child have a warm, loving relationship and that you have all the supports needed to keep yourself, your child, and your family safe, happy, and together.

# CHAPTER 4

# GET OUT OF DEBT
# AND STAY OUT OF DEBT!

This next step probably sounds like it has nothing to do with raising a disabled or handicapped child. In fact, most people might say that getting out of debt actually sounds harder than raising a disabled child. So why take on both of these challenges at the same time? Here's why this step is vital for you and your child's success and well being.

Having enough money to live independently means that you have more choices, control, and some level of financial security. Given the uncertainty that exists when raising a handicapped child, one thing you don't need is money problems. Also, remember we covered being different in the last chapter. Most families in America live paycheck to paycheck. Your life needs to be different than most people, so you have the flexibility, control, and independence to do what you need to do. This will reduce the stress you experience when dealing with your child's "special issues." Having the financial stability to do what's best for your child is empowering and allows you to feel good about doing all you can to help your child. Great, so we want to get out of debt. So how the heck do we do it?

My wife and I fell onto this secret many years ago, when I was traveling long distances back and forth to work. It's not really a secret, but boy it sure worked like one. As I drove to work each day, I happened to tune into a Christian radio station playing a broadcast by a man named Larry Burkett. Larry's program was focused on debt-free living, and it just happened to catch my interest. After listening to his program for a few weeks, I came home one night and asked my wife, "Hey honey, how'd you like to live debt free?" She said, "Sure." From that point forward, we began putting a plan together to pay off our house, pay off our school loans, and get completely out of debt. It was very difficult, uncharted territory for us. However, we actually pulled it off, and it totally changed our lives. Fortunately, we now have a better approach to get debt free for readers of this book. And this better approach is called the "Total Money Makeover (TMM)."

The Fox Business News channel has an individual named Dave Ramsey who has put together a wonderful program called the *Total Money Makeover*, which is a step-by-step program for getting your financial future in focus. Dave's program is a time-proven sequence of steps that, if followed one by one, will result in you getting out of debt and staying totally debt free.

Dave openly acknowledges that his program is based on the work of Larry Burkett and others—and he offers advice similar to what your grandmother would provide—but he says he keeps his teeth in. This part is debatable. (Smile.) However, his program packages and implements the step-by-step "get outta debt" plans in a simple, easy-to-do method, unlike anything else I've ever seen.

This program will totally change your life—and in the end, allow you to have the financial freedom, flexibility, and focus needed to properly raise your disabled child. One thing is for sure. Disabled children have unplanned expenses. They also add stress to your life. Imagine how much stress would be eliminated if you were debt free and had enough money to handle any emergency that came up for your child. Also imagine how you'd feel if one of the outcomes from raising your disabled child was that you got out of debt and were totally financially independent. This really can be one positive outcome from this situation. All you have to do is purchase Dave's book (*The Total Money Makeover*) and follow his recommended steps. It will take time, focus, and dedication to pull off.

You may not become a millionaire, and you may not make it all the way through the steps of his program. Your specific total money makeover may have to be adjusted to support the immediate decisions needed to help your child. But whatever progress you make will help you and your family members live a less stressful life. And it will allow you to fully love your child and do all you can to help their improvement by having the financial freedom to make whatever critical financial decisions are needed.

As mentioned above, we fell into this realization by accident, as I just happened to hear Larry Burkett on the radio as I was driving to work. I don't think this was an accident, as this totally changed our lives. However, we didn't have an easy-to-follow plan. Hopefully, using the total money makeover will enable you to make this financial change even quicker and more effectively than we were able to. We've raised our son for about sixteen years now—and have been debt free for about the same amount of time. Our house is paid for, and we have money in the bank. We also have five other children, all of whom have money saved for college. This stuff really works and *is* worth your time, effort and focus.  It will probably do more to help you raise your child than any medicine that has ever been developed.

In addition to doing your own total money makeover, there are also a wide range of other methods to help reduce the cost of raising your special needs child. Many of the special items you'll find helpful for your child don't cost much at all, depending on where you purchase them. If money is no concern, then you can just log onto www.flaghouse.com and see everything your autistic child will ever need. Flaghouse is a company that sells a very wide range of sensory and support items for disabled children. Their products are very high quality, and they provide very good customer service. For some of the special needs purchases you'll want to make for your child, you may have no choice but to order them from Flaghouse or a similar specialty company. Some items are so special in nature that they can not be found at other retailers. However, this is the exception, not the rule. Most items you'll need for the care and support of your child can be purchased locally. And depending on how handy you are, some can be made yourself. Just use good, conservative decision making when deciding these purchasing decisions.

As we tried to purchase early childhood development tools for our child (such as letter, cards, puzzles, and other early educational items), we found that most could be purchased at our local dollar store. Remember, your handicapped child will more than likely destroy any items you place in his or her span of control. So although it's wonderful to purchase the very best items, more than likely you'll be purchasing duplicate or replacement items on a continual basis. Unless you're related to Bill Gates, you probably will find that you'll have to budget your money. This will force you to prioritize what you buy and how much you spend on things. No surprises here.

Most dollar stores have a wide range of very useful coloring books, alphabet learning cards, number cards, and simple jigsaw puzzles. As the development process for your child will probably take much longer than it would for other children, these simple items make a big difference in terms of helping with development when working at home. I encourage every parent to work with their children to help augment what is done in school. For autistic children, the development and learning process is much slower and drawn out. So purchase simple, low-cost items that can be easily replaced.

Along with the normal learning items at these stores, we also found that our son needed some sensory stimulation aides. Of course we could have gone on the Internet and obtained these items from a specialty store. However, that would have cost a lot of money, and in the end most of these items didn't last more than a few hours. So we improvised, using items with similar sensory impact but at a much lower cost. Be creative and think about what you're trying to accomplish with your child. Consider your child's specific needs when selecting items. Finally, be sure to consider the risk of small parts, electrical shock, and other concerns when purchasing items to give to your child, just as you would for anything you're giving to a small child.

For example, you can purchase special vibrating or spinning sensory tools to help autistic kids mitigate their heightened sensory stimulation issues. These items cost hundreds of dollars at specialty stores. Instead, we went to a dollar store and found spinning battery-operated pencils, spinning lollipops, vibrating tooth brushes, and many other "sensory stimulation items" for about a dollar each. The lifespan of these items can be measured in hours, so expect to go through quite a few of them. However, don't rush out and buy them by the case. The specific sensory and developmental needs of your child will change over time. Sometimes special needs or behaviors will change rapidly. So assess what your child's needs are right now, then go and purchase the lowest-cost, safest method to make this happen. It's different for each child, but don't assume everything needed for your special needs child has to come from a special needs store or that it has to cost you an arm and a leg to get.

Early in the development process for our son we worked with an Occupational Therapist to help with his sensory overstimulation needs. We were taught how to properly brush our son and perform deep pressure exercises. I won't go into the details within this book, as you really need to be shown how to do this by a trained medical professional. However I'll briefly mention two things specific to what we learned about this early childhood sensory development technique. First of all, *never* brush the belly or stomach of your child. This causes significant internal problems and can permanently injure your child.

Second, the brushes we used for these exercises were given to us free of charge by our therapists. Even when we lost or broke the original brushes, replacements came at no cost. I mention this only because we thought about purchasing these special brushes before we were shown how to perform the activity. Once we got trained, we were given the equipment we needed free of charge. So wait until you know for sure that you need a specific item before you rush out and purchase the world. Most of what you buy is related to the timing of specific needs. As a result, stocking up in advance is probably only beneficial with respect to having enough diapers and wet wipes.

Another way we found to save money was on clothing. Remember I mentioned that our son shreds his clothing and will typically go through two or three sets of clothes in one day. I'm not referring to soiling his clothes; he actually shreds them. So there's no concern about having to wash most of them, just a need to continually replace them. This gets very expensive, to say the least.

We've adjusted our clothing purchases for our son to deal with this issue—in the lowest cost manner possible. First of all, we shop at Wal-Mart, and we're darn proud of it! We purchase the lowest cost jeans, stretch pants, and shirts for him, often buying ahead when items are on sale or on clearance. This helps reduce the ongoing impact to our budget. Another secret my wife uses is to purchase seasonal holiday clothing for him once it gets reduced down to 90 percent off. We purchased fourteen shirts for our son last week after Halloween was over. These normally cost anywhere from $5 to $10 to purchase. However, after the Halloween rush is over, these get marked down to 90 percent off or more. We got most of the shirts for $1 each, and a few for $0.50 each. Although it's only fourteen shirts, every bit helps.

I realize my son may not be the most well-dressed autistic child in the world, but to be honest, I'm happy if he's dressed at all. Most of the time he returns home from school in shreds of clothes that look more like torn rags than anything else. So when we look for clothing for him, the design, color, or brand name really isn't the issue. As long as it's his size, cheap, and not inappropriate material, we're good to go. Shopping cheap takes on a whole new meaning when you're buying the same kinds of clothing items over and over every day of the week.

There are some other ways to save money. Unfortunately, we didn't explore a lot of these, as our son's condition and care took most of our time to deal with. I've heard some very successful stories of parents saving a lot of money using coupons, joining discount bulk lot stores, and using other leveraged buying techniques. The Internet has a few coupon Web sites that are designed around making coupons easy to use, maximizing the discount and helping to organize your use of them. However, we simply didn't find these items the best fit for our specific set of circumstances. We went with cheap, clearance, after-holiday seasonal purchases in bulk when we could find them. I encourage everyone to explore as many options as you can to find creative ways to save money. Every dollar you save is one that can be used to better support your child and your family.

CHAPTER 5

# PREPARE YOURSELF, YOUR HOME, AND YOUR WORLD!

T his next step isn't something that is easily defined, but you'll know when you make this happen. Special needs children need special things around them. So don't be surprised if you find that raising them in a "normal home environment" or a "normal school environment" doesn't work. You need to put some focused energy on preparing yourself, your home, and your child's world to support these very special needs.

Preparing yourself means exactly what it says—prepare yourself. This may mean becoming familiar with your child's condition—by reading medical or other applicable material to help you understand your child's needs. It may mean searching the Internet for the latest forms of treatment, behavioral therapy, or other applicable items to help your child. It may mean taking the time to purchase and implement your total money makeover (remember, we're getting out of debt to help your child), which you would not have previously done.

Preparing yourself means taking some time, energy, and focus to do things that your child needs you to do. The key to this step is realizing that this requires your time and attention. When we went through this process, we found ourselves struggling to do all the "normal stuff" we used to do—but had these items competing with "other stuff" we needed to do for our son. So allow yourself the freedom and flexibility to become prepared for raising your special needs child. This will probably mean reading some materials you previously were not familiar with. It probably will mean engaging in some support groups or support materials that deal directly with your child's disabilities. It probably means making items a priority that previously you had not even thought about. Whatever getting prepared means for you is going to be specific with respect to your child. It's different for everyone. However, realizing that this step takes time, energy, and focus is important. Otherwise, you'll feel like you're competing with yourself for your own time. Getting prepared is important—and critical to provide the best care possible for your child.

Preparing your home is another very important step to ensure your child has a safe, supportive environment. I mentioned the Formica walls and ceiling coverings we had to install to help us address our son's "super-special" messes. Your family's special needs will be different depending on your child's specific disabilities. You may need to install special locks or other barriers to prevent your child from becoming injured. Some parents need to install special monitoring devices to ensure their child is supervised properly at all times. Others require special medical technologies to treat their child and support ongoing medical needs.

The list can be endless. However, keep your focus on your child's real needs for the moment, and your real priorities will eventually become clear. Home improvements cost money—and although we've taken steps to improve our financial situation, the funding isn't unlimited. So go with the items your child really needs right now, and prioritize them as you would any family investment. And remember, plan to be different. For example, we had to install keyed deadbolts on several doors in our home to prevent our son from wandering off. This looks a bit strange for visitors coming in, but it works very well for us. It wasn't expensive to implement, but in the end it turned out to be priceless in terms of the benefit.

Also remember that just as any child's needs change over time, your special child's needs will also change over time. What previously worked to keep your child safe may not work as he or she grows larger or older. Clothing needs may also change over time. Once we found our son had a tendency to shred his clothing, we purchased duplicate items. However, when we discovered him going through $300 worth of clothes in less than a month, we then had to go with cheap, disposable clothing to meet his "special shredding needs."

The next chapter deals with preparing your world. Assuming that you plan to try to raise your special needs child by yourself for the long haul (i.e., forever), then you need to realize one absolute fact. There are some places that are simply easier to raise a special needs child than other places.

For example, raising a special needs child on the waterfront may pose some very difficult challenges that may actually place the child in physical danger, depending on his or her specific disability. So carefully examine your child's short-term and long-term needs, as this may result in the realization that you need to relocate. This should not be done as a knee-jerk response or without careful consideration. However, one big thing to consider is the availability of external services to support your child.

Many states (such as Florida) have a very limited number of services due to the low tax base within the state. Alternatively, other states (such as Pennsylvania, Maryland, and others) have substantial support services available for special needs children. Also, within each state, the level of services is different by county, township, or local district. So where you decide to live can drastically impact the level of external support services you receive.

This is something to seriously consider, especially if your child has severe disabilities and would benefit from external support services such as behavioral therapy, vocational support, or special scholastic support activities.

CHAPTER 6

# GO AFTER SUPPORT SERVICES
# LIKE A BIG DOG! (WOOF, WOOF!)

Now that we've gotten past some of the basics, it's time to begin moving into uncharted territory. Assuming you've listened to our experience, you realize that there's no room for blame, your finances need a makeover, and the location you select to raise your special needs child is as important as how you raise them. So now what?

The real concern with raising seriously handicapped special needs children is that more often than not, they require more help than you or your family can provide. It's not just because they need constant supervision, infinite patience, or continuous love. In reality, special needs children need special help, often from professionally trained personnel. Simple learning tasks become infinitely more complex and take much longer when special needs children are involved. So you may think, *Okay, so I'll get some help for my kid—eventually.*

Ah, but there's the rub. The early childhood development problems of a special needs child require immediate attention. In fact, immediate intervention for an autistic or mentally retarded child makes all the difference in the world. So the next few chapters will focus on how to obtain that help—and how to get it very quickly and effectively. I'm not going to say it'll be easy. However, you'll have some shortcuts that should help you cut to the chase much earlier.

Many of the items listed from this point forward are generic in nature and do not represent the most current terminology, legal facts, or applicable programs for your area. In fact, it's likely that most of what I mention will be different when you actually do your own research. Rather than waste time trying to assemble a reference guide of boring (and immediately outdated) material, I instead will cover the principles behind getting services for your child. As you'll learn in later chapters, you'll have to do your own research, which will be dependent on your child's specific disability, the current laws in effect at the time you perform your search, the area(s) in which you live, and other specifics that you'll need to determine.

However, this won't be as hard as it sounds. This chapter will describe the very first step needed to engage in this process. Next, I'll provide some guidance not only on which services to go after, but also in which order. Finally, I'll provide a list of the tools, technologies, and other supports you'll need to tackle this head on.

One thing to remember as you embark on identifying and obtaining services for any special needs child: it isn't easy! No one (and no agency) will simply line up, ask, "So how much do you want?" and fill up your tank. It takes focus, determination, and some level of persistency. However, there are a few ways to streamline this process, and I'll do my best to clearly identify the best ways to achieve each goal.

Remember, your role is to become the best advocate for your child. It's unlikely that everyone you engage with (agencies, service providers, etc.) will come to the same conclusions you will. Nor will they likely offer the full level of services you feel would benefit your child. Be prepared to fight back—in a professional, persistent, respectful, and loving way. But never, ever give up!

Although there are many service providers who really do all they can to help these special kids out, more often than not, they're trying to reduce services, meet budget quotas, or eliminate services over time. So be prepared to fight for what your child needs—and ensure you use a few of the following tricks to help you win the war.

# KEEPING THE FOCUS ON THE HOCUS POCUS

erhaps the biggest impact to our lives was the requirement for supervision for our severely disabled child. This wasn't your typical "I gotta keep an eye on my kid" kind of supervision. It quickly became clear that our child needed constant supervision by qualified, trained, and responsible individuals, at all times.

You may think, *So what's so hard about that?* as there are lots of trained and qualified folks who specialize in caring for autistic children. Unfortunately, this simply isn't the case. There are many service providers who are ill-equipped to provide the supervision and oversight needed for kids with the most extreme cases of autism. And given the severity of our child's condition, few people on the planet had any idea how to properly supervise our child—including us! Of course we had the normal "care for the baby night and day" responsibilities at first. However, as things progressed and our child got older, we found that our son wasn't physically disabled. As a result, he began exploring his environment just as any other child would.

As our son began to develop his cognitive, sensory, and emotional disabilities, it became very difficult to maintain control over him. Although I'm hoping that most folks reading this book will not be faced with a child with this severe level of disability, I am covering this subject for those who are faced with the same, "So what the heck do we do?" kind of situation.

Our experience was (and is) at the far end of the spectrum, when even tears, prayers, medicines, and professionals can't help.

The first thing we found was that our son would often endanger himself, even in a tightly controlled environment. He would put inedible items in his mouth, bite himself, cut himself, and injure himself whenever we were not directly monitoring him (visually) and controlling his actions. I recall one night when he was about four years old, being in the family room with him. I was watching him closely, while he was playing on the floor. I happened to be on the phone speaking to my relatives; however, I was focused on watching him closely. In less than a minute, he climbed up on the sofa next to me. I thought he just wanted to sit next to Daddy, which was fine.

However, as he climbed onto our L-shaped couch set, he stood up on the sofa and in a flash, ran all the way around the sofa. That wouldn't have been a problem, except he never stopped when he got to the end of the couch. He fell headfirst into the end table and split his bottom lip wide open. My amazement was only interrupted by my shock as I saw him run, fall, and start bleeding all in a matter of about three seconds. I threw down the phone, called for my wife, and then we rushed him to the emergency room. I felt terrible, as if I had done something wrong. However, as the years went by, future experiences of this type made it clear that this child would endanger himself no matter how much control was placed over his environment. So it's vital that anyone watching him be prepared, qualified, and responsible enough to handle this task. At the time this event occurred, I wasn't prepared, and he showed me quickly how unprepared I really was.

One of the most important things to remember when raising a disabled child who needs this level of supervision is that you cannot just assume that a professional understands the needs of your child. In our case, we could not assume anyone (even ourselves) could be prepared to handle the things this child could dish out. I recall another time when we took him to his special school. Of course we had met with the school program director and had set up a dedicated aide and other special supports for our child. We were sure they knew he had to be supervised at all times and reviewed the types of events he had experienced, so there was no room for doubt.

"It'll be fine," they said. "We deal with these kinds of children every day," the program director assured us.

*Okay,* we thought. *We've written down and discussed his special needs, got a written contract with the school regarding the dedicated aide, discussed previous events, and well, of course, we're dealing with professionals who do this all the time. We're probably worrying for nothing, right?* Wrong! About three weeks later we got a call saying they were rushing our son to the emergency room, as he was choking on something but they had no idea what it was. When we got to the emergency room, the school teacher said they thought he had inhaled an eraser off the end of a pencil. However, they just were not sure.

How could they not be sure, as didn't his dedicated aide see what was going on? That's when we were told his aide wasn't in class that day. I won't get into the reasons why the aide wasn't there, as everyone knew this was required in his specialized plan. I also won't mention what was discussed next with them. However, the point is that in some cases you can't trust anyone to understand the complexity or severity of your child's needs. No matter how hard you try, prepare, document, and communicate your child's "at risk" behaviors, it's very difficult to ensure that everyone supervising your child will understand the magnitude and complexity of the situation.

While we're on the subject of school, make sure you clearly complete all paperwork regarding the transportation of your child, including any special transportation needs. The law requires that children with special needs be given an appropriate education, including safe, reliable transportation. On the form we completed, there was a question about, "Can your child be left unattended when brought home?" Heck no! Not only can our child not be left home alone when dropped off, he needs a dedicated aide, special restraints, and other supports just to go for the ride. Try explaining to your family why it's so hard to come down for a visit when you're faced with requirements like this just to send your child to school. It'll make your mind spin.

Okay, enough about school. Let's talk about other supervision requirements at home. Babysitting is another effort in futility. We tried to find suitable candidates to watch our child for many, many years. They'd all start out the same way, saying, "Oh, I'm sure it'll be fine" or "I have a grandson with special needs" or "I'm sure it's not as bad as you say." Well, all their good intentions ended with a horrified look with them running out of our house yelling, "You need a priest. This child is possessed by the devil!" Our response was always the same. "Okay, thanks, we'll call you if we need you again. Take care." (Smile.)

It quickly became obvious to us that we needed to tightly control who was supervising our child. School placement became a very complex and rigorous task. Babysitting only became possible after years and years of teaching our other children how to handle our son's condition. However, for about the first twelve years, it was up to us. Our relatives could not help us, as none of them could even imagine the supervision requirements for our child. So my wife and I partnered together, supporting each other in this task. We prepared ourselves, our home, and our world for making this happen successfully. And I'm happy to say that in sixteen years of watching him, aside from the initial couch event and few smaller surprises, our son never got seriously injured while under our care. Notice I say "while under our care," as we did have several other surprises while he was at school.

Remember when I began this book I said that it was written to try to help those parents who are faced with the most extreme cases of this type. So I realize that some of you may disagree with what I'm about to say. But that's okay. If your child doesn't have this severe level of disability, then God bless you, and do what's needed for your specific child. However, if you have a child as bad (or worse) than our son was, you may find that your life isn't your own anymore, in terms of how you spend your time. We'll deal with the subject of time management later in this book. However, for now, I think it's proper to prepare yourself mentally for what your special child's supervisory needs will do in terms of your life.

I hope you're raising your special needs child in a partnership with someone you love (i.e., your spouse or significant other). It's not that I believe that all families need to have two parents, or that the conventional family is the only method that works. My statement is simply that a seriously handicapped child can dish out more than one person can handle. If you don't believe me, come on over and watch our son for a full day. We've had that offer on the table for quite a few years, and he's challenged even the most attentive professional staff. So you need to realize that many of the things you previously did for yourself (such as free time, going out, sleeping regularly, etc.) may have to be put on hold until your child either stabilizes, improves, or is placed permanently in the care of others.

Given the serious nature of the potential injuries a child like this can suffer, I seriously recommend that if you're a single parent trying to raise a child with this level of illness that you find someone you can partner with to help with these responsibilities. Raising any child alone can be very challenging. However, raising a seriously autistic, mentally retarded child with cognitive, sensory, emotional, and possibly physical disabilities by yourself is impossible. You simply can not handle all the needs of your child alone. So whether it's a close family member, special someone, or whoever, get the help before it reaches the boiling point. Otherwise, you'll be in crisis situations and trying to get help at a time when no one is able to understand the complexity of the situation. At that point, you'll need as much help and assistance as your child will need.

Anyone who is trusted to watch your child needs to have the right disposition, training, and dedication. For special needs children, there's also two other requirements. The first is having the patience of Job (this reference is from the Bible). Special children take time to do even the simplest of tasks. They often make mistakes. They also regress or lose the skills they've previously been taught. Teaching them to improve takes years, and sometimes never is successful. It takes a special kind of person to give them the love, patience, support, and acceptance they need for success. This is one of the reasons I feel that a single parent cannot raise the most extreme cases of autistic children themselves. I just don't think anyone is that patient all the time, 24/7, 365 days a year, at all hours of the day and night, for many, many years. Not me anyway. So if you think you're up to it, I suggest you write a book showing others like me how to do it.

The second requirement is knowing how to discipline these kids, using positive reinforcement. Normal discipline doesn't work on these kids, as they don't understand what's occurring and cannot process normal verbal feedback. Spanking these special kids is totally insane and out of the question. "Why?" you may ask. "My dad spanked me and I turned out okay. If you spare the rod you spoil the child." I am not suggesting that you do not discipline your child in any manner, but this is what we experienced as we tried to get our child under control.

Many of the emotional and physical outbursts of our son were completely beyond his ability to control. For many years, I thought, *What a horrible, evil child,* as he'd try to hurt others, hurt himself, and break everything in sight. However, as we learned more about our son's condition, we realized that his brain had specific sensory, cognitive, and emotional imbalances that could not be corrected, even with medication. His world, his perception, and his self-control were all very different from what a normal child experiences. Many of the items he ripped, destroyed, or threw were the result of his brain being on overload, with no other release available for him.

So we realized that the only way to discipline or control our son was through the use of positive reinforcement. Positive reinforcement is a method in which you reward your child for behaviors that are acceptable. For a severely autistic child with these disabilities, behaving acceptably may be something as simple as going to the potty, not ripping up a book, not shredding his clothing, or some other task that you may initially think is no big deal. For autistic children, it's a very big deal. And if your child does what you want (and controls inappropriate behaviors) then you provide an appropriate reward.

Rewards can be anything from giving your child a favorite toy to play with, allowing some time off from drills, or of course, providing food rewards. We initially had to begin with food rewards, as they were the only thing our son responded to. For him it was beef jerky, as he loved the stuff. We'd ask our son to do whatever we needed him to do (or not do). "If you clean up the mess on the floor, we'll give you some beef jerky." His response would be to pick up one item, then come over to us with that big, wonderful grin we know and love, and ask for "beef turkey" as only our superman can do. This was much better (and more effective) than yelling at him to clean up the mess and then trying to spank him when he didn't do it properly.

Food rewards are probably the most effective in terms of getting results. However, longer term, you'll need to switch the focus from food rewards to other, non-food reinforcements. Giving candy, beef jerky, and other food-related treats to special needs kids can result in them becoming seriously overweight and can cause other health issues. So do what's needed initially to get your system of positive reinforcement going. Then work longer term to switch this to a non-food based system of reinforcements. I'd also suggest you write down the positive rewards and reinforcements that work for your specific child. This will help others who provide supervision to know what works best for your child as a means to control specific problem behaviors.

Positive reinforcement can also be reversed when your child is misbehaving. Just as with any child, you can withdraw enjoyable items as a means to guide inappropriate behaviors. Taking away their TV, favorite toy, or other pleasurable item is a way to let your child know, "If you're good, you get this. But if you're bad, you will lose it." This may seem obvious, but remember, many of these kids are non-vocal and significantly mentally delayed in terms of their comprehension. So it may take a few times before they catch onto the fact that you're not just being mean.

There's really a method to the madness, and eventually they'll catch on. This doesn't mean they'll always do what you want or behave. However, they will understand that this event is occurring as a result of their behavior, which is a huge accomplishment. Timeframes may be extended, results may not be 100 percent, but the process will be in place to allow you to discipline your child when they misbehave. And you won't be trying to spank your child, which will make things much worse.

So how could spanking a special needs kid make things worse? What could be worse than an out of control, severely autistic child who is ripping up clothing and smearing poop on the walls and ceiling? Here's what's worse: a child who learns that he should hit himself or others when things go wrong.

This is a fact that we learned through observation and monitoring our son. He learned through direct observation of his environment and by listening to others (as auditory processing was his best skill). So if we yelled, he yelled. If we hit, he hit. If we got out of control, he also got out of control. It was sort of a monkey see, monkey do kind of situation. This is how most kids learn. However, autistic children cannot get the additional feedback, experience, or benefit from the discussion that normally accompanies these kinds of events. They simply experience it in their own unique way. This means they try to imitate what they've experienced.

We had one caregiver who obviously was hitting our child, although we never saw her do it. Our son began hitting people after being under her care. He'd also mimic some words he must have heard her say. "You are bad," he said, and he began hitting himself. This quickly demonstrated to us that we needed to do two things.

First, we got our son away from this caregiver, permanently. Second, it showed us that we needed to be very careful how we disciplined our child and what we exposed him to. Otherwise, we'd be inadvertently teaching him some things that we never intended to do. He could develop very inappropriate responses to everyday experiences, which we may have no ability to reverse. So how we reacted to his "special messes or out of control outbursts" became as important as any other aspect of his care. This was especially critical when he was young, before he developed his limited speech abilities.

I realize it's very hard to maintain control, be patient and loving, and react the "right way" when you're faced with some of the challenges these special kids can unleash. I recall one day I came home from work and found our son had thrown his diaper all over his room. It was on the ceiling, walls, floor, him, us, everywhere. We spent the next four hours steam cleaning his room from top to bottom, just so we could put him to bed. I was exhausted.

We cleaned him up, got him ready for bed, took him to the potty, and said goodnight. About half hour later I went in to check on him. Guess what I found? He had done the same thing all over again, with poop everywhere. I just about blew a spark plug in my brain and my initial response was … well let's just say it was not optimal. However, I immediately remembered that this child was very sick, not bad. He really couldn't control himself and was just engaging in the world around him in a manner as best he could. My wife and I spent the rest of the night cleaning things up again.

Although I have to admit I was ticked off and not thrilled with our son or our life at the time, we didn't spank our child. Nor did we teach him any additional bad behaviors. We actually had him help with the cleanup activities. This was obviously a closely monitored activity, and to our surprise, he indicated that he didn't like doing the cleanup. After a few more episodes like this with us making him help with the cleanup of his mess, he stopped making these messes completely. We did exactly what we needed to do. However, I've got to admit, it was very hard not to react per my initial gut response and drop kick him into our neighbor's yard. (Smile.)

'This level of self-control needed by the parents is a skill that takes time to develop. For us, the breakthrough was the realization that our child was very, very ill, not just being bad. Had he been missing an arm or a leg, I think it would have been easier to realize just how sick he really was. However, from the outside, he looked normal. So it was something that took a lot of internalization and time for us to learn so we could care for him with the type of controlled responses that were needed.

Working together with your spouse, significant other, or close family members, it's important to realize that you eventually need to take a break. Depending on the circumstances, your health, and other specifics, the frequency, quantity, and duration of breaks will be unique for your own specific needs. The title of this book, *Raising Superman!,* references the fact that these kids are special, and their needs sometimes require super-human response levels. It's also a reminder that despite all the love and support you offer them, you can't do everything alone. None of us are that superhuman, and even the best of us need some help at times.

# THE SPRINT FOR SUPPORT SERVICES

The first step we found that got things rolling was to contact our local branch of the Mental Health/Mental Retardation service provider. Their number was listed in our local phone book under "MHMR—Mental Health/Mental Retardation." This agency can help you to identify services applicable to helping your child's early and long-term development needs as well as provide some other family support services.

They won't just pick up the phone and say, "Can we take your order?" or deliver your request in thirty minutes or less, like a pizza. You'll need to call, identify yourself, clearly describe your child's special needs, and respectfully request a case manager. Let me repeat this. Request a case manager. You may ask, "Why do we need to ask for a case manager?" Because you *need* a *case manager!*

Setting up the correct programs and support services for a special needs child requires the experience, skill, and support of a competent case manager. We had a wonderful one who really helped kick things into high gear.

She came out to our home and visited with our child. I'll never forget the day she came out. She called to tell us her name was Roz, and after speaking to us about our concerns, she said, "Don't worry. I'm sure it's not as bad as you describe." Then when she got to our home, our son was playing in the family room. We offered her the face shield so she could go in and "observe him." She turned to us and said, "That's okay, I'm sure I won't need that." We both looked at each other and thought, *Okay, well* **she is** *the professional.* Once she went into the family room, we heard her say, "Hi, Norman," and then all hell broke loose. We heard growling, parts breaking, and then we saw papers flying out of the doorway. The case manager came running out of the room, all out of breath. She said, "This child is horrible and needs to be institutionalized immediately!" We simply smiled at her and said, "Roz, he's actually having one of his better days."

At that point, we sat down and obviously had her full attention. When the day was over, she provided an amazing amount of help. She informed us that our son would qualify for a medical access card as a result of his disability. This was vitally important, as it opened up the door for him to receive a wide range of services, which he normally would not receive under our private medical insurance. In fact as I understood it, all disabled/ handicapped children automatically qualify for medical access as a result of their disability, regardless of their parent's income level. She helped us complete the department of public welfare (DPW) application and expedited the processing of it. So if you're faced with a similar situation and do not have your child enrolled with MHMR or within the DPW Medical Access program, make that priority one!

Once we verbally requested the medical access card for our son, the department of public welfare sent us the official application. This next part is extremely important when applying for public assistance/medical access for any disabled child. Although the forms and application package you are completing ask for your income statements (which you still need to provide), you must put on the top of the application package (and any forms) that you are applying for a disabled child very clearly. If you put this statement on the top of the application package and on any forms you're submitting, then your request for medical access for your child should be approved, regardless of your income level. Do not forget to put this on all of the form(s)! Also do not assume that you do not have to submit your income information along with your completed application. Any missing information will delay the processing of their medical access card, which costs you time, requires effort to correct, and delays receiving the services that are badly needed by your child.

Along with the medical access card, our MHMR case manager also informed us of other services that would benefit our child. Another service she helped us set up was a diaper service for our son. This allowed us to order any size disposable diapers he needed and have them shipped directly to our home—at no cost to us. This is significant, as part of our son's autistic condition was accompanied by chronic diarrhea. Unfortunately, she didn't last long once we got this initial meeting over, as I think she was possibly fired for doing such a great job with us.

We spoke to the medical doctors about this aspect of our son's medical condition, and all we could conclude was that some autistic children have constant chronic diarrhea, but no one knows why. All we knew was that he went through about ten to fifteen diapers a day. This adds up, and unfortunately, since he remained in diapers until he was about fourteen years old, the cost and quantity of adult-sized diapers continued to expand exponentially until it was bigger than anything imaginable. The diaper service was a blessing from heaven and allowed us to focus our remaining funds on other needs for our son.

Initially when we enrolled our son in the medical access program, we were included in another program called HIPP. This program reimbursed our family for the cost of private medical insurance for our son, as opposed to having us use medical access for all of his medical needs. Eventually this program changed into an HMO-type coverage, which replaced the HIPP program reimbursements. I encourage each of you to check into the current medical coverage options for your disabled child, as I'm certain that the options available for you will be different than they were when we first enrolled in the program. However, two things are vital to remember.

First of all, your child needs medical insurance even if you think the rest of your family doesn't need it (or can't afford it). The medical coverage for disabled children should be provided at no charge by the state (or you should move to another state). In addition, their medical needs are much more significant and continuous than any normal child. So trust that you'll need this coverage for both medical and behavioral treatments. And expect that you'll use it often. That's the first vital thing to remember.

Here's the second. Never (ever, ever) maintain two sets of medical insurance for your disabled child at any time, under any circumstances. Having medical insurance coverage is mandatory. Having more than one medical insurance plan is death by appeal, as neither insurance company will pay for the bills and you will be caught in a continuous circle jerk. In the event that your child has existing private medical insurance and you now qualify for medical access (and assuming you're not covered within the HIPP program), immediately notify your private insurance carrier to drop the coverage for your child effective on the date that you have confirmation that the new coverage goes into effect. Do not let the two plans continue together, or you'll be very, very sorry you did.

The only exception to this statement is for those enrolled within the HIPP program. The HIPP program requires you to continue your private medical insurance and instead of receiving benefits under medical access, you are reimbursed for the portion of the cost of your private medical insurance related to the portion covering your handicapped child. So for HIPP enrolled participants, you will need both plans (private medical coverage and MA/HIPP). However, this is the only instance I know of where having two plans works.

We encountered this situation when my son's medical coverage was moved from the HIPP program to the standard HMO insurance plan (funded through the state medical access program). We thought, *Great, we'll keep his old insurance just in case the new insurance doesn't pay something.* What we got was a runaround and continuous notices from both carriers that his "other primary insurance" should pay. So in the end, neither insurance company paid for the pre-approved services. Finally when I went to cancel the one insurance, I had to fight to prove he had the other insurance and almost had to wait a year for our work "open enrollment period" to cancel this other coverage. Do yourself a favor. If you get the HMO type Medical Access Health Insurance for your child (which should be at no cost to you), then immediately cancel any private or other medical insurance they have once you have verification that the new coverage takes effect. You'll thank me in the long run.

One final comment before we move on. There are some case managers (such as the one we initially got) who are worth their weight in gold. I truly believe that these folks are not paid enough for the high-quality service and contributions they provide. However, for every good case manager, therapist, or specialist, there are probably ten bad ones. These other people are definitely paid too much for the crappy service they provide. And it's up to you to distinguish between these two extremes of service providers.

So the message is pretty simple—expect and demand to get these services set up quickly, effectively, and completely. Don't let anyone tell you, "There's a waiting list," as that's not your problem. Getting your child into a full-time care facility may require being on a waiting list. Getting your child set up with medical access, diaper services, and a case manager should not put you on a waiting list. If it does, just jump to the chapter on the power of print and you'll know what to do. Otherwise, be polite, demand to know how long things will take, and if their response involves looking at next year's calendar, then you know you're getting hosed. Applications for medical access for a disabled child should be completed and submitted within a week, processed and approved within three to five weeks, and services should begin no later than two months after submittal.

Remember, you can always request a new case manager—and we did this several times. Unfortunately, as you'll find out, the work lifespan for these case management individuals (especially the good ones) is measured in months or single years at best. So it's likely that you'll have several case managers as your child grows through these programs. However don't settle for a bad one. You'll know if you have a bad one as nothing happens but you get continuous promises or explanations as to why you're requesting something that's not appropriate.

Also remember your child's development is at stake, so push for what's really needed to address critical special needs. Demand written guidance on the programs, and take the time to read the material to become familiar with it. Learn the escalation and appeal processes. Be your child's best advocate and demand the very best. Getting prompt and proper services early for your child now might make all the difference in terms of becoming self-sufficient later in life.

CHAPTER 9

# LET'S RAP ABOUT WRAPAROUND

At this point I need to make an assumption before I proceed. This will impact the priority of the items you need to go after for your specific child's needs. I'm assuming your child is too young for school, and you've been fortunate enough to read this book shortly after your autistic or handicapped child was initially diagnosed (ages between two to three years old or younger). If this is the case, then there is another type of service you should investigate for your child. These services are called "wraparound support" and involve the support of a Behavioral Services Consultant (BSC), Behavioral Specialist (BS), Occupational Therapist (OT), and Therapeutic Support Staff (TSS).

A BSC is an individual who comes into your home and develops a program for your child to begin accelerating early childhood development and address specific developmental needs. This sounds very "medically oriented"; however, it essentially means setting up wraparound services, which can include the LOVAAS/ABA drill programs, which we found very helpful for our son. These drill programs are a structured method in which delayed or autistic children are taught how to process learning new information. It's a long, tedious process, involving hours of "drill time" done in the home by a TSS and monitored by the BSC.

Although the drill programs are long, tedious, and somewhat annoying, they really work. It won't take your child from being significantly delayed to a point of being a rocket scientist overnight. However, for my son, who was incapable of learning anything new, it taught him his colors, numbers, basic letter recognition, and helped him begin to speak more clearly. I don't want to mislead anyone on the success rate of these activities, as our son's drills took years to perform. We also had a few secrets I'll share on how we "improved his results." However, this program did a lot for helping our son improve at a very early age when we thought he was essentially un-teachable. In addition to the educational and learning benefit to these drills, the program also began to teach him a bit of self-control, anger redirection, and other internal control skills. This wasn't a magic pill, but it did help a great deal over the years during which it was implemented.

So depending on the severity of your child's disability, you should seriously consider implementing wraparound services, including the LOVAAS/ABA drill programs using the support of a BSC/TSS. In addition to the drill programs, we also had wraparound staff to work with our son and play with him during the week in the evenings. They would play with him in the yard, take him outside for walks, try to teach him to ride his bike, and generally try to provide a companion for him to safely monitor and help with his development—up to about sixty hours a week of services initially. Longer term, the services were reduced as our son improved and no longer needed this intensive level of wraparound support. However initially, these services were vital for his success in our home. And remember, this was all free through the MHMR case management services and billed under his medical access card.

Once we had our son's program in place, we immediately began to see the pressure to reduce our son's service benefits. I mention this only because every parent receiving these services gets the same pressure. First they give you sixty hours. Then they tell you he's only approved for thirty. Next they'll tell you that they can only fill twenty due to having no staff. And so forth and so on. So don't fall for it. All programs such as these require tight and consistent documentation of progress. The agency will need to collect and document your child's progress from the drills, so get this information from them. Become familiar with it, and then use it to fight to maintain your child's service levels.

Remember, you are the best and only advocate for your child. If your child needs these services, no one will fight hard for your child's benefit except for you. So don't let some budget quota take your child's future away. In most cases, the true benefit from the LOVAAS/ABA drills occurs within the first four to six years of doing them. So these service levels won't be this high forever. However, the timing window is short so ensure your child gets these services as soon as needed. Don't settle for delays in getting services; escalate concerns if needed. Finally, don't settle for service level reductions; escalate and fight these as needed.

CHAPTER 10

# LET'S TAKE A RIDE!
# SPECIAL TRANSPORTATION SUPPORTS

This next chapter covers a few things we were totally unfamiliar with in terms of special supports my son and our family really needed. Some of these items I felt kind of ashamed to use, but over the long term I learned why we qualified for these items. I encourage each of you to consider whether or not your child and family would benefit from these supports, and if they are needed, go for it. Don't worry about what other people think or the fact that many of these services are sourced through the department of public welfare. In many cases, these services are really addressing a special need for your family and help keep the care needs for your child minimized in terms of expenses.

When we initially met with our case manager from MHMR, we learned that we could apply for a handicapped parking sticker for our son. This seemed strange, as our son didn't drive and probably never would. So I questioned whether this was appropriate for our son to have, as none of our other family members were disabled, handicapped, or faced with limited mobility.

It only took a few "close calls" for me to realize that not only did our son need the handicapped parking access for his safety, but that we also needed it for our sanity. Our son was a really difficult case to transport. In many instances, it took us about thirty minutes just to get him into and out of the car. Once we arrived at our destination (which was normally a hospital, doctor's office, or service agency), we had to closely control his exit so he could safely make it into the building. On several instances, he darted away from us and almost ran into oncoming traffic. On other occasions, he'd drop to the ground, having one of his severe emotional outbursts. Needless to say, having a parking location close to our destination was vital in terms of our ability to safely transport him.

Now I can't tell you how many times we got "weird looks" from people who saw us park in these handicapped parking spots. I'm sure they thought that we were taking advantage of the situation, especially on the few occasions where our son got in and out of the car with little effort, walked quietly into the building, and sat down, acting as if nothing was wrong. These days did happen, but more often we had some kind of unexpected, significant outburst or challenge from him. How do you explain to a seventy-year-old lady who comes up to you and says, "That's just not right!" when you park near a doctor's office in the handicapped space? All I could think to say was, "You're right, lady, he's not right in his head." However, this really didn't accomplish much.

So we learned to bite our tongue and just ignore most of the comments. Occasionally someone would say something I just couldn't ignore and I'd wind up informing them that the only thing worse than my son's condition was their insensitivity and ignorance to the special needs of a severely autistic child. However, all that did was make me feel better at the time; it really did little to address the situation. So in the end, ignoring the comments was just easier. Learn to live with these kinds of comments, as it's par for the course.

Other services are available to transport your child to and from medical appointments if needed. You should check with your case manager to see which services are available in your area. The key here is that your child may have unique special needs requiring special supports for transportation. Use these services if there's a real need. Be thankful and appreciative that they exist. But don't feel guilty about using them, as these services are provided to address behavioral and medical needs, which few people fully understand.

Doctor's offices may or may not be prepared to fully deal with the level of difficulty your child can create. We've been thrown out of many offices when our child went into full tilt mode. On other occasions we were quietly asked to leave. I recall one time we flew in a plane to go to a specialist office in another state. I won't mention the airline carrier, but once the doors on the flight closed and the air pressure changed, all hell broke loose. The pilot gently asked us to take a different airline for our return trip and handed us tickets for the other carrier. How's that for subtlety?

I highly suggest you prepare any offices that are scheduled to receive you in advance so that you can maintain a healthy relationship with them. For example, our son had a very limited timeframe during which he could be kept waiting in any office environment. Sometimes doctors can be late for their appointments, especially when it comes to specialist appointments. I highly encourage you to inform your doctor's offices of any difficulties that may arise from keeping you or your child waiting longer than expected for an appointment. Make these notifications in advance, prior to your arrival at their office. And let them know the significance of this issue so they are really prepared.

In some cases, it may help to have them take down a note to call you in the event the appointment is delayed prior to your arrival. In the most extreme of circumstances, you may want to ensure the office knows the maximum time you'll be successfully able to restrain your child in the event your appointment(s) is delayed. Some professionals will understand and appreciate this feedback. Others may not. It's only possible to try to be as proactive as possible as you prepare for taking your severely handicapped child out into the world.

Remember, when it comes to autism, many of these children look very "normal" and show no outward appearance of any problems. This causes a lot of difficulty when it comes to others understanding the level of complexity, difficulty, or sickness your child is faced with. We struggled with this for years and often felt that had our son been missing a body part or been hooked to a respirator, he would have gotten much more support from others. Instead we were often ridiculed for allowing him to get into the shopping carts while we forced our other children (which just happened to be girls) to walk alongside him. "Oh, what's the matter? The boy is too good to walk?" we'd hear. "Can you please control your son? You need to discipline him!" we were told by one of the store managers. Or my favorite was when the store manager came up to me and told me that I needed to spank my child and that I had no idea what being a parent meant. "Okay, buddy, you know best," I said back with a smirk. "I'll get right on it."

The point is that you'll never get the understanding or support from others that you need to easily deal with your child's issues. So don't expect to. Just realize that special needs kids are special and that most people have no clue what you're up against. You can try to inform them, print out cards, play an audio tape, make a speech, or get ticked off at them. Eventually you'll realize this is just part of the routine, so ignoring them is probably about the best that you can do. However, there are a few of us out there who do understand, and when we see you, we'll give you a big thumbs up!

# CHAPTER 11

# BELIEVE IT OR NOT, SCHOOL IS A BLESSING!

This next chapter is very important, as most of your child's development and improvement may result from specialized school-based programs. We've already prepared the family for all the "special things" your child needs to have in place. We've met with our case manager(s) and completed as much early intervention support as possible. We've improved our financial situation by trying to limit costs and get out of debt. Finally, we got the handicapped parking sticker and other transportation related services needed to safely transport our child. Now it's time to discuss school placement and the development of your child's individualized educational plan (IEP).

Our familiarity with the next few items is based on our experience for our son and our other children as they became eligible for school services. One interesting fact about raising an autistic child is that their impact in the home environment often causes developmental problems or delays for other children in the home. Said another way, having one child with autism may cause your other children to exhibit some specific types of developmental delays. In our case, it was obvious that our son being in our home caused our other children's speech and motor development to become delayed. Their delays were not nearly as significant as those of our son. However, in each case we needed early intervention services to work with our children to correct these developmental delays.

What we found as we worked through these issues was that our local school district had a wonderful program for assessing the needs of pre-kindergarten aged kids and placing them in programs to address these specific needs. For our kids, the services were provided by the Lincoln Intermediate Unit. This program picked up our pre-kindergarten aged children at our home, worked with them in a structured setting providing speech, occupational therapy, and other services, and then returned them home each day. This was a wonderful program, and it really made a difference in the early development and recovery for our children. Also, these services were free, with no charge to our family. In my opinion, these services are vital for those families needing them, and I know for us they made all the difference in the world.

So how do you engage in these school-based services? My suggestion is to contact your local school district and find out who you need to contact to have your child thoroughly assessed in terms of a full-range skills assessment. The school district should set you up with a date and time to bring your child in for a comprehensive battery of tests, including speech, cognitive, sensory, and other types of evaluations. Your child will be interviewed and assessed by a panel of experts who will document the range of skills (or delays) your child exhibits and make formal recommendations for special placement or services. The assessment should also be accompanied by a series of hearing and vision tests, although I must admit that interpreting the results of these tests is difficult.

How do you interpret the lack of response by a three-year-old autistic child to a vision test when they don't speak, can't focus, and will barely sit in the chair? In many cases, the results may indicate that the test was inconclusive as to whether your child has hearing, vision, or other issues. However, it should help in getting prompt placement into a proper setting to begin a specialized educational program.

In my experience, all of our children with developmental delays followed the same general process, with our son's process just having more complexity. This basically means that all our kids had an individualized educational plan (IEP) developed to address their specific needs. The IEP program is very specific, with processes, procedures, and guidelines defining what must occur. Parents must participate, and I highly encourage everyone to be closely involved with all the decisions being made that impact your child. The development of your child's IEP will impact the goals, services, and outcomes you can expect throughout the school year. So it's important that you understand, comment on, and agree with the decisions made. If not, you'll miss being the great advocate your child needs to ensure he or she is as successful as possible long term.

I won't take any additional time in this book to describe the specific IEP processes we went through for our kids. The process changed yearly, and the guidance, requirements, specific forms, and services available also changed from year to year. Instead, I'll just recommend that you call your school district, ask about the early intervention services, have them set up an appointment, and send you any written guidance on the engagement and assessment processes. Once you meet with them, you'll begin to learn more than I can communicate about the specific programs available in your area. And as I've mentioned earlier in this book, if you find that your specific area has few or no programs for your special needs child, then seriously consider moving. We found the services in our local area to be a critical part of our success in raising our severely autistic child, and we could not have been successful without these services.

As your child transitions from early intervention services to regular school-aged placement, you may find that you have some difficult decisions to make. For example, do you homeschool or not? Do you have an in-school aide for your child or not? Do you have your child taught in your home as opposed to going into the school environment? I'll briefly touch upon each of these subjects so you can at least get my opinion as to what worked best for us. It's okay to disagree; however, please take heed of the cautions I list, as you could easily forfeit some of the benefits your child may get from school.

Let's discuss homeschooling for a moment. I realize that many people currently home school their children. And they do so very successfully. Many families do not feel that public or private education outside of a homeschooled environment provides the right control over the academic environment to properly guide their child's development. And for those folks who feel this way, then I commend and applaud all those who homeschool their kids, as it may be the right choice for you.

However, our situation was just a tad different. Our son ate rocks and twigs. He pushed holes in our drywall and tried to put the insulation down his pants. It was obvious to us that many of the benefits of homeschooling were just not applicable to his situation, as he could not understand or relate to many things. For our son, it was about putting him in a safe environment and getting him the speech therapy, occupational therapy, and other programs needed to stimulate his development. Early on, we didn't even understand what these programs were, let alone do them ourselves in the home. So homeschooling wasn't appropriate for our son.

So now we knew he had to go to public school, and we were involved with the development of his IEP. Next, the subject of an in-school aide came up. Should we use a portion of his wraparound hours to have MHMR provide an in-school TSS/Aide, or do we require the school district to provide their own aide for his safety while he's in the classroom? Hum ... seems like an easy question and no big deal. Either way would work, right? He has a great wraparound aide now working with him at home, so why not have these same services in school to supervise him?

Now pay attention to this next response, as this is very important. Under no circumstances do you ever mix service providers when it comes to developing a program for your child. Put another way, if the school needs a primary support aide, then the school needs to provide one. Of course the school will tell you that his wraparound support would be the best place to get his aide for school. And of course, his wraparound supports coordinator will tell you that the school needs to provide their own aide. In both cases, each service provider will try to put the cost of the dedicated aide on someone other than their own budget. However, the cost of these services is not the issue.

If you agree to have the primary in-school aide provided by your child's wraparound services (or via any other service provider), then you may be letting your school district off the hook—forever. They have no responsibility or obligation to obtain the aide for you and will simply look at you and say, "There's no aide for your child so you need to get to work on providing one through your wraparound service provider." Huh? I thought the school had to set up the programs, ensure the safety of our child, and provide the required transportation for them? Sure they do, but only if you require them to by what you agree to in your child's IEP.

So be very careful what you agree to when working through the details of your child's IEP. Don't fall for the statement of, "Well, let's try this and see if they need more services." Also, don't put your child's safety at risk. If your child needs a dedicated aide in the classroom or on the bus to maintain continuing safety, then demand that this be added to the IEP. *Do not compromise on safety needs for your child!*

Remember, these special needs children are unpredictable, and even the most competent trained professional staff can be surprised by them. Overlapping, defense in depth support is needed to ensure they remain safe at all times. If agreement cannot be reached during the IEP meeting, do not sign off on it. Demand to be given the written escalation and grievance process. Execute the escalation and grievance process if needed. Remember, you are the best advocate for your child, and you know best regarding their needs. Others may be more familiar with the school programs, but not more familiar with what's best for your specific child!

Finally, I want to offer a comment on performing school instruction in the home. We had this offer made to us on several occasions, when it became challenging to transport or maintain control of our son in school. I do not recommend that anyone allow their school district to bring a teacher into their home to complete the requirements of educating their child. Here's why.

First of all, we found that the best part of school was getting our son out of the house. We realize that this was difficult for his bus driver, aide, and teacher. However, having him home 24/7 was more difficult. Getting him out of our house provided us with a desperately needed break so that we could take care of the tasks associated with raising a large family. While our son was away at school, we were able to complete our shopping, clean his room, do his laundry, and all the other items we could not do while we were continuously watching him. This may sound like a trivial issue, but trust me, it's not. Getting a break for us by sending him to school was one of the major contributors to our overall family's success in raising him.

The second and more important reason not to allow your child's schooling to occur in your home is that the number and level of service hours will not be identical. This isn't a widely known fact, so please pay attention to what I'm about to say. When your school district established your child's IEP, they have specific goals that need to be met. Often, these goals are targets, and it may take years before progress is made.

The school district may offer to bring someone into your home to implement your child's IEP and work toward accomplishing specific goals. However, I'd be amazed if they'll commit to a high number of in-home teaching hours each week. And if they do commit to a number of hours, it'll be far less than the amount of time your child will spend in school. Realizing that the bus ride and lunch activities add to the duration your child is away in school, you may find that in-home instruction only occurs for three or four hours a day, and possibly not every day of the week.

So unless you're compelled to want to keep your child in your home environment permanently and allow the school district to provide a smaller number of hours for your child's education, I highly suggest you send him or her to school and not allow the instruction to occur in your home.

I do want to pause here and say that our school district was eventually wonderful to work with. They helped us obtain some very significant services for our child and listened to what we thought was needed for his safety. When things didn't go well, they spoke to us as real people, and we worked through the challenges together. In the end, it is a partnership, so don't get the impression that it's all just one long battle. However, it may take them some time to realize that you mean business and that you won't settle for seconds. Once you've established what you think your child's needs are and they realize you are not leaving until these are met (assuming the demands are reasonable), then they should be willing to work to implement the appropriate services with you for your child's success.

# CHAPTER 12

# OTHER SPECIAL SUPPORT PROGRAMS TO CONSIDER

Forgive me for what I'm about to say, but I almost entitled this chapter "Becoming Relentless." The intent of that statement is that many of the services I'm about to describe are very difficult to enroll in, set up, or receive services from. However, if your child's needs are significant enough to require these additional supports, then I suggest you go for it. However, expect to have to get your game face on and have the tenacity of a professional vise grip. Also expect to experience biblical levels of delays, stall tactics, and other methods to wear you down. It becomes a battle between good and evil. And when it's over, you just won't know which side is which.

There are several programs called "waivers" you can enroll your child in based on specific needs. Some of these programs, such as the person family directed support waiver (PFDS), will actually provide you with funds that you can direct to spend in a manner decided by you and your family. Naturally there are restrictions on what is appropriate for purchase under the program, and it takes a lot of tenacity to apply for, follow up, get approved, and finally be successful at using this program. However, this is another way to pay for the specialized equipment, services, and other supports your child may need.

An easier service to engage in is the use of family-driven funds (FDF). Family-driven funds are another program run within each local mental health/mental retardation agency. The intent is to provide families of special needs children with a smaller amount of financial support for specific purchases critical for their child's success. For example, the PFDS waiver may cover purchases costing anywhere from one thousand to five thousand dollars. Family-driven funds would normally be used for purchases costing less than a thousand dollars. So although the two programs are different, have different enrollment requirements, and provide different levels of financial support, both programs can provide additional sources of funds to help raise your autistic or special needs child.

Another service to consider is vocational support services, once your child becomes a bit older. Vocational support services do exactly what they sound like. These services are used to help prepare your child for some type of vocation or work-related activity, with the intent of becoming self-supporting long term. In our specific case, it wasn't something that would benefit our son, as his specific disability makes him so unpredictable that work vocations are not an option for him right now. However, many children significantly benefit from this service, as it helps prepare and equip them for long-term employment, despite their significant special needs. Again this is dependent on the specific circumstances, cognitive level, and emotional stability of each unique child or adolescent.

We have not talked much about the benefit of many of the external support groups for autism, so these are absolutely worth mentioning at this time. The National Autism Society does a great job of disseminating information that can be very helpful when raising an autistic child. Your local chapter of the NAS may also conduct meetings and seminars or send out newsletters to keep you informed of things that may impact your child.

We initially went to a few meetings local to our area and found that the biggest benefit from attending was the networking done with other parents. Although we're a private family and don't like to share much in terms of our confidential issues, we found that other parents were a wealth of information we really benefited from. So my suggestion would be for new parents of special needs children to attend at least a few support meeting in your local area to speak to the other parents and get as much out of their local network as possible. Once you've done your initial meetings, you can decide if there's a longer-term benefit to your continued participation in these meetings.

To be honest, we found that after we attended our initial meeting, most of the other meetings were not applicable to our son's needs. Most of these meeting were focused on the school-based transitional issues for older kids, and our son simply wasn't old enough to benefit or be impacted from these items. It was nice to know about, but we had other challenges at the time that required more direct attention by us. So we didn't continue to attend these support group meetings.

However, the initial benefit from going to the first few meetings was intense. We learned about the wraparound services, the IEP program, case management, ABA drills, and a wide range of other items that became vital for our son's success. I want to thank all the parents who share this information freely, as it's been one of the best means for new parents of special needs kids to come up to speed quickly. It's also one of the reasons our son was able to get the help he needed as quickly as he did. And for that, we're forever grateful.

CHAPTER 13

# PROTECTING THAT WONDERFUL, INNOCENT SMILE!

arlier in this book we discussed medical coverage, health needs, and a variety of other items that directly impact the well-being of your child. I thought it would be helpful to cover the dental care aspect of your child's needs. Keep in mind that it is possible that an autistic or special needs child may be able to go to a normal dentist. It depends on the severity of their condition and the reaction to things that occur at the dentist office. Sometimes, things can go well. I'm actually trying to say this with a straight face, as you probably know what's coming next.

If you're faced with the serious nature of what we experienced with our son, there's no way a regular dentist was ever going to get anywhere near our child. It was obvious that our child needed a "special dentist" for his "special needs." What I'm about to review are some of the basic things we learned regarding dental care for our son.

First of all, our son had to be put to sleep for all dental activities, regardless of how small these were. This wasn't obvious when we initially tried to get his dental care set up. Our insurance companies made us "try to do things in a step-by-step fashion" and would not immediately agree to put him to sleep for the procedure. So we began by taking him to a specialty dentist who tried talking him through the procedure. You know how that went. It was a total waste of time.

Then we were given some liquid medicines to try to make our son drowsy, so the dentist could get his job done. This was another huge waste of time. No dental work was done, but our son was extra cranky the rest of the week. Finally, when all else failed, we were successful in convincing our doctors, insurance providers, and health plan that our son needed to be put to sleep using anesthesia for his dental checkups and for all dental work. In hindsight, the first few attempts to do this with the liquids and other items probably were needed, given the higher cost and potential reactions that could come from putting him to sleep. However, it took the better part of a year before any dental checkups or fillings were done on him. So be prepared for this tangled web of delays and medical bureaucracy.

The other item I want to mention is to make sure you know what your specific out-of-pocket costs will be prior engaging in any services, including dental work. Make sure you get any out-of-pocket costs identified in writing prior to approving or engaging in these services. And finally, shop around if they are unreasonable.

The dentist we initially went to said that they charged several hundred dollars just to put our child to sleep in addition to what our insurance would pay. They also said that they were the only dentist in our county that performed this kind of work on autistic children. They lied to us. We found several other dentists who performed the procedure with no out of pocket costs being incurred by us. The other dentist we finally went with completed this procedure in a local hospital setting, using the latest form of anesthesia and monitoring equipment.

This experience showed us that we needed to confirm our out-of-pocket costs prior to agreeing to any services and take this into serious consideration as we selected our service providers. Don't just accept that your insurance won't cover all costs—check around before making a final decision. It also showed us that not all the information we received from service providers was always accurate. This is something you may want to remember, as it could help you at a later time. We would often get told that our insurance only covered 80 percent of the cost of the service. I'd review my dental plan and it showed that we were covered at 100 percent, or that my son's dental coverage would be picked up by his medical access card. "Oh yeah," they'd say. "You're right—we were looking at the wrong form, or the wrong benefits schedule."

Challenge what you're told when it's going to cost you money, and know what your policies cover. You should be able to easily get a schedule of benefits from your service provider or insurance company for your medical and dental coverage. Use these as your defense against improper charges, as you'll find there's several ways to pay more than you really should owe. Hum ... people lying to us in order to get our money. This isn't something specific to raising an autistic child, but certainly is a good thing to watch out for.

# CHAPTER 14

# THE POWER
# OF PRINT

This chapter can be summarized in one sentence. If you are ever told no to a request for your special needs child, it only means you have not pushed hard enough. I'm going to cover the basics of becoming a super-advocate in this chapter and share some of the secrets we learned throughout our years of struggling and doing battle with the various agencies. Of course, your experiences may differ and you may find you have no use for these tips and tricks.

Yeah right, and Santa Claus is coming down the chimney. Take good notes as we go through this material and mark the chapter so you can find it over and over again. (Smile.)

The first thing to remember when engaging in services for your child is that all programs have a basis in written guidelines, policies, and procedures. In fact, if it's a government program, there's probably more material written describing how the processes work than you could ever imagine. In many cases, we found that our service providers had little understanding of what was actually documented regarding their own processes or programs. You can and should demand the overriding process, policies, and guideline documents for any program or service you wish to engage in be sent to you. Also ensure you ask for the latest revisions to be sent, along with any other applicable materials, forms, or submittal documents.

You'll be amazed at how few service providers will be able to easily produce this information. However having the "real facts" about how any program operates is critical for negotiating through the tangled web of bureaucracy that exists when you apply for support services that cost real dollars. In some cases, you may get lucky and services may be provided on the first try. But eventually, you'll be turned down. And remember, being told no simply means you have not pushed hard enough. So expect this to be an iterative process, with you applying, appealing, and appealing again, many, many times. Remember, good things are worth fighting for.

Also make sure you know your rights as a participant in any program, service, or process you're engaged in. Many processes have a patient bill of rights or other document defining exactly what your rights are, what your child's rights are, and what process you can follow if things don't go as expected. Request to get a copy of your rights as a participant under each program you're engaged in. Keep these documents organized so that you can refer to them. Check the date or revision level of these documents prior to using them. And get revised copies if these documents have been updated since the last time you've used them.

The next item is pretty basic, but you'd be shocked at how few people realize this fact. Everyone has a boss. You have a boss. I have a boss. The head of our local MHMR has a boss. In some cases, the boss of the agency directors is a state or federal official. However, it's still their boss. And bosses can be contacted when their employees don't do what's needed. Don't be intimidated by anyone who says, "I am the boss." This is crap—and don't fall for it. Everyone, regardless of position, has someone they report to, or some body of people accountable to ensure he or she performs appropriately. Escalate items as needed to fight for what your child needs. And although I don't recommend you escalate everything immediately, once you've given the normal process time enough to work, get moving up the food chain.

I'll share one example we went through to raise this point. Our child required a very special environment to protect him from injury. I'm sure you get that by now. We had a deck attached to our home that sat about thirteen feet above the ground. Our doctor and case manager agreed that our son could endanger himself by climbing over the three-foot-high railing and could fall, seriously injuring himself. So we approached our case manager to see if there could be some family-driven funds to help pay for a higher railing to protect our son.

We got the typical runaround. First, they lost the request. Then they said that there was no money left for the year. However, we were told at the beginning of the next financial year, they'd consider the request. When the next year rolled around, they said this request was not acceptable to pay with family-driven funds, and the circle jerk went on. I finally got ticked off enough to call the boss of our case manager, and then the county administrator for MHMR. I may have also called a few levels higher, as it's been some time since this happened, and I forget the specifics.

However, I eventually got to someone who would not help me and I said, "So who do you report to?" "That would be the state governor," she said. I thought she was lying to me. "You're telling me that there's no one you report to between you and the governor?" I said. "Yep, that's correct," she replied. "Okay, can you please give me their number?" I said. She did, and I called the governor's office. To my shock and amazement, she wasn't lying to me—but regardless, I wasn't getting what I needed to keep my child safe.

I called the governor's office and left a voice message informing them of the serious nature of the safety issue endangering my severely autistic son and the runaround I got for the last few months. To my amazement, I got a return call within the hour. The governor's office worked this issue with me and provided a funding source and the approvals for installing our safety railing (which turned out to become safety walls). I mention this example not to brag or suggest that you immediately call the governor's office for all of your child's needs. However, the point is that everyone reports to someone who is accountable for their performance. Don't be intimidated by their position, authority, or tone. They put their pants on each day just like everyone else.

I also want to communicate the point that there's more than one way to skin a cat, or in this specific reference, more than one way to fund a need. We had originally asked for family-driven funds to provide the safety railings needed to protect my son. Although I believe this was appropriate in terms of the funding source, the governor's office identified a different "pot of money" that was made available to us to fulfill this need. Maybe it was to protect their agency's reputation? Maybe it was because FDF were not the right place to fund this? Who knows? In either case, it doesn't matter. We got the funds we badly needed to protect our child from falling, and they got to address this need in the manner they decided. Everybody won. But it was a long, hard fight.

The power of print works in both directions. What I mean is that you should certainly obtain and read all the process, policy, and guidelines applicable to any process you're engaged in. It's your Bible when it comes to fighting for the things you need for your child.

However, you should also submit your requests in writing if you expect them to be taken seriously. There's a lot of power in the printed word, even if it's you who wrote it. You can certainly try to make your initial requests verbally, as I know writing letters takes time, effort, and follow through. However, we quickly learned that in most cases, verbal requests were somehow ignored, lost, or misrepresented. As we got more experience in effectively working through the "system," it became obvious that real requests needed to be submitted in written form.

Sending in written requests does a few things. It clearly documents what you're asking for with respect to services for your child. It allows you to clearly document the need-based request and send along any supporting medical documents verifying the applicability and appropriateness of your request. Finally, it allows you to establish a timeline during which you can begin to expect responses. Most government processes have timelines for expected responses written into their policies. It's not okay for an agency to get a written request and sit on it for six months and then tell you they never got it. Send your requests along via the U.S. Mail, with a return receipt signature requested. Keep these return receipts as a means to verify that they got the request. Build a steady, consistent source of information documenting your request and all responses to date. You'd be amazed how much a little organization and documentation will do toward getting you the escalation and approvals you need for success.

There is one other thing I'd like to mention while we're fighting for our children's needs. Don't feel ashamed or sorry that you're taking things to this level for results. It's to be expected. Remember, in the end you'll only get things approved if you continue to escalate and fight for things using the appropriate appeal processes. You'll only have to win one time to realize that the delay game is meant to wear you down. The longer these requests take, the less has to be spent. It's always about the money. However, if your request wasn't valid, you wouldn't eventually win, would you?

So put this to the test. Apply for something your child really needs. Submit that request in writing. Follow the applicable process guidelines and see if it's approved the first time. If not, don't give up. Appeal, file a grievance, or do whatever is appropriate for the item(s) you're requesting. Continue to fight. If your experience goes like ours did, after about three to four appeals, you'll be given the approval to proceed for your child.

Finally, do not withdraw an appeal, complaint, or grievance without having an official written response from the agency you're battling saying that they're doing whatever they agreed to, if you hear them say it verbally. Verbal statements may not be binding and are very hard to prove. So do not let them manipulate you by telling you one thing and then going back on their word. Agencies have e-mail just like the rest of us, and it only takes a short amount of time for them to send out written confirmation if they sincerely intend on doing something. We made this mistake one time—when we were told to withdraw our complaint, as the request had been approved. Fool me once, shame on you. Fool me twice, shame on me! Don't fall for it, as it's one of the oldest tricks in the book.

The next thing to make sure is that you understand any timelines associated with the processes you're engaging in. For example, many requests for services have timelines associated with them for appeals on decisions. If you miss the timeframe for appealing a decision, you forfeit your rights to the appeal process. It's imperative that you know all the timelines and appeal processes as you send in requests. Otherwise, you'll only be able to get approval for the most basic services for your child and a wide range of more complex (and more expensive) services will be lost.

Expect for most of your requests to initially be rejected. Plan to have to appeal at least two or three times before the more substantial services are approved. Don't get discouraged or let anyone make you feel bad about doing this. Know the processes by reading all applicable process documents. Set dates on your schedule so you're prepared to respond to any hearings, appeals, or responses ahead of the due dates. Keep good records and expect to have to follow up as needed. Be the super advocate your child needs to fully develop his or her untapped potential.

Now I want to speak directly to all the fathers of these special needs children. I'm not being sexist, but I do think the following statement is true. Fathers have one of the most vital roles to play as families work to do the very best for their special needs children. I'm not suggesting that moms are not just as important. It's just that fathers do have some kind of special impact on the response families get when applying for services, dealing with their school district, or engaging in struggles to keep services. Here's why I'm saying this.

When my wife and I began our adventure in trying to get services established for our son, it became painfully obvious that I got a better response than she did. Initially I wasn't sure if it was because I handled these situations better, or if in fact men were treated differently. I'm sad to say that it's the second—men are in fact treated differently when present at these meetings. Or at least, that's been my experience to date. Perhaps it's the impression that's conveyed when both parents show up at the table, indicating a fully involved and loving family. Perhaps it's the working professional at the table, taking time from his busy schedule to participate in the needs of their child. Perhaps it's the threat of being sued? Who knows? All that I can say for sure is when I'm there, things go better. I've seen this with other families as well. In my experience, a mother coming to the table to fight for her child's services will have a much more difficult time negotiating than two parents side by side or a father leading the charge.

It's okay if you disagree or call me a sexist pig. I know this is a bit controversial, but if it works, we're going there. I'm telling it like it is. I'm simply offering this "opinion" (which I think is a fact) so that you can more easily obtain, set up, and keep all the services needed by your child. Oh yeah, and one more thing.

*Dads, don't be absentee owners with respect to these activities.* Otherwise, you'll be letting your spouse, your family, and worse, your special needs child down. You really have a special role to play in all these items. Even if your heart's not in it, your mere presence will help when meeting with the county agencies and school district. If you don't believe me, try it both ways. Then you can judge this for yourself. You'll quickly see what I'm talking about just by the responses you get at the table. So be there and stay involved!

Remember the beginning of this chapter was about never giving up. If you're told no to a request for your special needs child, it simply means you have not pushed hard enough. That being said, also make sure you pick your battles. Some items will absolutely be critical for the health, safety, and well-being of your child. Those items you need to fight for. Other times, you may "need" an item, but you may not feel it's worth going to battle over. Remember that every escalation has some level of consequence associated with it, so pick your battles wisely. However, if you know your child needs an item or service, and it's appropriate to request under a specific program, then I say go for it! Just remember, you can't hit the "escalation button" every day. Use it when it's appropriate, and your child will really benefit.

Do not give up or become frustrated if these processes take a while. Be honest, open, and polite, but do not expect things to just happen all by themselves. People will not just provide support because they're nice. You'll need to fight to keep your child's place in line for these services. Always keep the live discussions professional and be certain that you are presenting yourself as an advocate for your child. In most cases, you'll be the only one fighting for what's right for your child. So it's no wonder why your opinion may be different from others at the table.

Remember, funding is limited. So expect to have to fight for the needs for your child. Stay focused, be professional, and keep informed of any process changes. Request meeting minutes or summaries of verbal discussions. Challenge what's being told to you and look for hints about the overriding processes, policies, or guidelines covering the requirements for the process you're engaging with.

Another trick I learned over the years was to use a third-party point of view so that emotion is removed from the equation as I fought for my child's services. This is pretty simple to explain, but takes a bit of skill to actually do. When you're engaged in an emotionally draining, highly charged battle for your child, pretend in your mind as if you're doing this for someone else's child, not your own. This may allow you to focus on the facts, real needs, and rights of the child without bringing all the emotion, sensitivity, and previous history into the discussions. Act as if you're a third-party advocate for your own child, and work diligently as if you were doing this for a friend. It may allow you to see some additional opportunities or allow you to regain control of an emotionally charged battle.

However, at the end of the day, this stuff does take an emotional toll on you. So prepare yourself, become organized, read up, and get that printer fired up. As we became familiar with the processes I was often called, "The guy who wrote the letters." Agencies hated getting contacted from me, as they knew I'd take things as high as I needed to in order to properly obtain services for my son. I didn't always do things correctly, and a few times life overtook our battles, so I had to let things drop. But all things considered, our son promptly had all the services he needed, which helped his overall development. That's about all you can hope for, if you do everything correctly.

CHAPTER 15

# DR. SPOCK
# VERSUS DR. SEUSS

W e will now touch upon some of the most controversial information in this book, the medical "stuff." Remember as you're reading this material that I'm not a doctor, nor am I a medical professional. I cannot offer medical advice, so please use a great deal of conservative decision making before deciding if any of the suggestions, conclusions, or approaches mentioned in this book are right for you or your family. I highly encourage you to discuss any treatment methods with a qualified medical professional before taking any action. And of course, please consider that all special needs children react differently to medications, treatments, and procedures. So don't make any rash decisions.

As a final disclaimer and to be perfectly clear, I do not want anyone to try any of the items listed within this book, for any reason.

There, that should put the lawyers out of a job. One thing we found early in this endeavor is that in many cases, our doctors may not know what's best for our child. Many of the professionals we saw either had very little useful information for us, or they prescribed methods of treatment that were totally ineffective for our son's specific condition. It took us a while to realize this, and our hopes were only exceeded by our dreams of making our child "normal" again. However, despite our continued search for a magic bullet, we found that conventional medicine had little to offer us.

We did try what felt like thousands of treatments, medicines, and other techniques to try to make our son better. Although we didn't have any success on most of these items, I highly encourage each of you to seek out any and all forms of treatment that could potentially benefit your child. Discuss these with your child's doctors and any applicable specialists. Finally, try them with appropriate levels of medical supervision to see if they work on your child. There are many instances of children who have a miraculous recovery from autism if the right form of treatment is applied. This doesn't mean that all children with autism can get better overnight. Nor does it mean that every condition can be treated. However, you never know until you try.

Many parents have had a great deal of success in using diet control for treating autistic symptoms. The standard more widely known version is a gluten- or wheat-free diet. Other parents have successfully cured their children by using dietary supplements, screening for internal intestinal diseases (Candida), or by looking for hormonal or enzyme deficiencies. The list is probably endless, and despite the fact that you need to carefully examine which of these "miracle cures" might be right for your child, in the end a devoted parent has to try. If for no other reason, just to ensure they've left no stone unturned.

I'll share our own experience with the secretion enzyme to make this point. We had tried a variety of miracle cures for autism, including a special diet, enzyme supplements, medicines, and other forms of treatment. One day we were watching the TV and saw that some parents had cured their autistic children overnight using an enzyme called secretion. We were very excited, and inside we probably felt as if our son was one shot of secretion away from being cured overnight. So we contacted our doctor to see how we could get this treatment for him.

Unfortunately, the use of secretion for treating autism isn't approved, and there are very few doctors who will perform this procedure. However, it is an enzyme used during upper gastrointestinal investigations (upper GIs) to activate specific processes inside the digestive system during investigative medical procedures. As our son had chronic diarrhea, I asked if we could request an upper GI (using secretion, of course) to determine the cause of his chronic diarrhea. This was approved by our doctor and our medical insurance. We were set! The procedure was scheduled at a very famous medical hospital in our area. We were very excited. We could almost taste the improvement our son would make once he got this vital enzyme given to him. The procedure was given, and he received the secretion.

After the procedure, nothing changed. Our son was still autistic. His behaviors didn't improve. The doctors were unable to verify the cause of his chronic diarrhea, and in the end, we went on with our lives pretty much with everything unchanged. However, we slept a bit better knowing that we had at least confirmed that this would not miraculously cure him. Otherwise, we would have wondered our whole lives whether we missed the magic bullet. The chances of this working for him were slim to none, and we knew that inside. However, the need for us to try this was as real to us as his autism, in terms of the emotional impact to our family.

We also tried the whole gamut of medications that are the standard battery of tools used by modern science against autism. We tried Adderall, Ritalin, Lorazepam, Seroquel, and about a hundred other medications. My personal opinion is that none of these medicines did much to improve our son. Each came with a wide range of side effects, additional behavioral changes, and mood outbursts, making it questionable whether the cure was worse than the disease. This may not be the outcome you see for your specific child. Depending on the severity of autism and other metabolic specifics, you may find that something like Ritalin does help. However, our experience wasn't typical, and modern conventional medicine apparently had nothing to offer us.

I previously mentioned the success of our son's drill program, which was basically a behavioral therapy training program. This provided huge benefits, not only with respect to teaching my son some skills, but also in terms of measuring what medical changes were effective. We observed the following as a result of his drill program, giving us our first clue as to what medicine would really improve our son's condition.

After performing our son's drill program for several months, it became obvious that his progress would be very slow. He took months to learn new items, and he often regressed or forgot new information. The process was very painful to watch. One day while I was walking through our local Wal-Mart, I saw a bottle of memory enhancement supplements. Specifically, these were products that contained Ginkgo and Echinacea. I asked my family doctor if these could be safely given to our son. He replied that we could try a small amount, and it should not hurt him. So we tried.

Now here's where things got interesting. We gave our son one tablet of each of these supplements over a two-day period, one Ginkgo, one Echinacea. He went totally out of control, with emotional outbursts and violent mood swings. This was about typical for him when we tried other medications, so we didn't think much more about it. We immediately discontinued use of these supplements.

But then, something unexpected happened. Our TSS came down that week and said our son had moved ahead three lessons, which was incredible. He appeared focused, alert, and had demonstrated greater ability to retain new information. *Hum,* we thought. *Could this be related to the supplements? Ah,* we thought, *but we've been down this path before.* As my wife and I discussed what had occurred, we both agreed that although our son had exhibited an improvement from these supplements, the dosage appeared to be way too high. *How high?* I wondered. Could this child be so sensitive that even the smallest amount of supplements would have a positive effect? Could we titrate his dose to allow him to see the benefits from this substance without causing the mood swings and violent reactions we had seen so many times before?

We had to try.

So I took our coffee maker and heated up a pot of water. I diluted each capsule in approximately one cup of warm water. Next, I put these solutions into a dropper bottle, and proceeded to give him four to ten drops of these solutions in a small cup of soda over the next few days. The results were amazing! His cognitive abilities improved dramatically. Drill performance also improved. The TSS and BSC kept asking us if we had given him smart pills. At the time, we didn't volunteer what had occurred, as we really wanted to see if there was a measurable, unbiased improvement in his performance. And it was obvious that this occurred.

Now I want to balance what's being said here with the reality of the situation. This supplement formula didn't cure our son of autism. He is still heavily autistic, and has all the violent behavioral tendencies associated with the condition. However his memory, ability to process, and drill performance all rapidly improved (almost overnight). What's also pretty incredible is that the amount of the supplements he received was so small that I had trouble believing that this small amount of natural herbs could make such a difference. But it did!

Now we were onto something. We knew to pay attention to the little things. Although some medicines caused a significant reaction within our son, we knew that we could measure his drill performance to see if any of the medications prescribed for him provided any real benefit with respect to his development. As we continued the use of the Ginkgo and Echinacea supplement solutions, our son began to acquire the ability to speak. In fact, we've often been told that he's one of the few children with this severe level of autism who can speak and communicate verbally.

I attribute this success to the work we did with the herbal supplements. Without them, he could not even begin to retain new information. Eventually, he would plateau, and he became stagnated. We tried increasing the supplements, but it did not provide any additional benefit. However, we did find something that actually helped, and we got this treatment to our son in time to allow him to learn to speak. Oh, what a success!

There was only one other time we found something that helped our son improve, besides the herbal supplements. This occurred when he came down with an ear infection. We came into his room and he kept yelling, "My ear has a boo-boo, my ear has a boo-boo." We looked but didn't see anything wrong. So we took him to the emergency room to have him checked out.

Without going into a long story, I'll simply say that the emergency room doctor looked in his ear and said, "I see an eyeball." "Huh?" we said out loud. "What do you mean you see an eyeball?" The doctor proceeded to use a small tool to go inside our son's ear, as we held him down to the table. To our amazement, he pulled a complete dollar bill out of my son's right ear. Apparently our child had stuffed an entire dollar bill in his ear. So much for the reason he had a boo-boo.

I swear, you can't make this kind of stuff up. And no, the dollar bill didn't make him any better. (Smile.) However, the emergency room doctor suggested that we put our son on some antibiotics to prevent him from getting an ear infection. *Okay*, we thought. *Why not? Maybe it'll help when he sticks the rest of the change in his other ear.*

So we put him on some antibiotics at our doctor's request. He had his typical reaction, getting very moody, violent, and out of control. But then we saw a dramatic improvement. His eyes were able to keenly focus on ours. He continued improvement of his learning and progressed even further on his drills. Finally, his ability to control his self-injurious behaviors improved dramatically. Again, this wasn't a magic bullet, and our son did not miraculously recover, but he did show signs of serious improvement.

We discussed this improvement and thought, *Could we perform the same type of low titrated dose using these antibiotics as we had done using the herbal supplements?* The answer was yes, and we performed the same basic process—one tablet diluted in about one cup of warm water. We gave him about the same number of drops. The results were staggering at first. His behaviors significantly improved. He began using more complex speech. His sensory sensitivities appeared to decrease. However, this only continued to a point. After a while, he stagnated.

But the facts were clear that certain substances in very low doses were able to positively improve our son's performance. Over a period of several years, I scoured every piece of medical information I could find and eventually I found a way to prevent the stagnation and plateau effect that occurs over time. However, nothing we've found will make him totally recover from his autism. It only allowed him to regain control over his most significant emotional sensitivities and outbursts, develop the ability to speak, and respond to verbal commands. Not a miracle cure, but certainly a big improvement!

I mention these items not to suggest that you try this (or anything of this nature) on your child, for any reason. Our experience was accompanied by the involvement of our doctor, specialist, and other professionals. Certainly no one should do anything without the involvement of a qualified medical doctor. However, for our son, nothing helped. We discovered these items by accident over years of trial and error, and by performing our own research when things stalled. And I'm putting this information into this book so that someone may benefit from our experience.

Perhaps this may lead someone in the research field to finally develop a cure for autism. Or maybe it will help others find a treatment that works long term for the spectrum of autistic disorders. Either way, this is what we experienced. And although it was an unapproved, unorthodox form of treatment, these were nonetheless the beginnings of two very successful forms of treatment..

Remember, special needs children can have negative reactions to medications and supplements more often than they'll experience positive benefits. Make sure you consider all the outcomes before allowing your child to undergo any treatment, use any medication or take any supplement. After all, the name of the game is to make them better, while ensuring their safety and well being at all times. This takes some time, effort, and key observations skills.

However, if your experience is like ours, you'll eventually see something happen that may improve your child's behaviors. I challenge you to carefully determine what that was, and how you can benefit from it. See if you can leverage it even in the smallest way to help your child improve. It may be short term or it may be a permanent cure. But in either case, any improvement helps.

# REFLECTIONS
# IN THE MIRROR

I thought it might be useful to take some time to actually describe the various behaviors, actions, and nature of our son's condition for those folks who really have never been exposed to this severe level of autism. It may be clear from the previous chapters just how difficult our son was to raise. However, until you've lived and loved someone close to you with severe autism, it's difficult to comprehend the full spectrum of what this condition does to someone's life. It is also impossible to predict exactly how far a child with autism will progress, as every case is unique.

From the years of discussions with our specialists, one thing became very clear. Autism is a spectrum disorder, with instances ranging from very mild cases to the most significant types. Every child is different, and therefore every case of autism has some unique problems or issues associated with it. Our son unfortunately had one of the worst cases of autism the doctors had ever seen. Had we not been fortunate enough to discover a few herbal supplements and other items that helped with his development, it's likely he would have continued banging his head and being totally non-verbal his entire life.

To get things started, I'd like to reinforce the fact that having autism from the outside means that the person looks perfectly normal. Initially, there are few signs that a young child has any problem at all. Aside from the crying that took place when our son received his initial shots, he seemed perfectly okay. However, as soon as his normal development began, we found that he wasn't progressing as we expected. His crawling just didn't happen, despite our family trying to work with him. We also found that he would regress or forget items we had previously taught him. Then the emotional outbursts began. He'd scream uncontrollably, laugh for no reason, and mumble sounds we could not understand.

At about three years of age, he became very violent and impossible to control. He would also try to hurt others who would come to play with him. I previously mentioned the use of a face shield when we would play with him. This wasn't a joke, and I was not exaggerating. It was very difficult to engage with our son, even for happy play time. He would try to grab, pinch, poke, or do anything to hurt others who came near him. Toys were instantly destroyed, as was our home. The house we had scrimped and saved for became a total disaster area, with holes in the drywall, messes on the carpet, and broken fixtures throughout the house.

We always realized that our son was sick, not bad. However, I have to honestly say that many times I was very mad about the damage he caused. My wife and I had many long discussions about what to do, and what not to do. We could not punish him in a conventional way, as he simply did not understand. It was also painfully obvious that the hitting, throwing, and other outbursts were beyond his ability to control. His sensory system was on overload, and nothing we found would help calm him down. He was very unpredictable, and as a result we had to quickly adjust our lives to keep him in a safe, controlled environment.

I know this is difficult to read, and probably more difficult to understand. Our son's condition impacted the lives of everyone in our family. We were unable to travel, and spent most of our free time searching for ways to help him. Work became another complication. In the end, my wife became a stay-at-home mother to attend to our son's needs and the needs of our other children.

Although I worked to support the family, I turned down many promotions and new offers, as these didn't line up with the needs of our family. I had to ensure I was close to home, as raising our child typically required two full-sized adults. He would often go into a full tantrum rage, kicking and screaming while thrashing around on the floor. It took both of us to hold him down. Our fear was only equaled by the tears of sadness that filled our hearts every time this occurred. We could barely look at each other. For a long time, life seemed pretty horrible.

Taking our son outside our home was (and still is) very challenging. Often, we'd get comments from outsiders when our son would react to something in his environment. "Can't you control him?" they'd say. Or "If he were my kid, I'd spank him," others would say. None of them had any idea of the sickness this child was suffering. And as we worked through the years, it became more and more obvious that few people, including professional medical specialists, had any clue as to what this child or our family was going through.

Remember, autism is a spectrum disorder, so there's more children with autism that are "better" than our son then there are who are as bad as him. Each case is unique, which is why I'm hoping that many of our readers will not have to suffer the misery we went through. However, as I promised in the beginning of this book, I'm not sugar coating it. My intent is to help as many families as possible by sharing our experiences, especially the things that helped. Each and every improvement was significant for him, our family, and our future.

There were three main ways that we could externally see our son's condition. These were through his facial expressions, outbursts, and his eyes. His face was either displaying intense sadness or joy. There were no mild emotions coming from him. He'd break into tears or laughter at the drop of a hat. We tried for years charting his behavioral mood swings to see if there were triggers or specific items that would set him off. In fact, many of his behavioral specialists and doctors asked us to repeatedly perform this same task and chart his outbursts. What we found was that there were no detectable trends in terms of what set him off. It appeared to be totally random. Or if there were specific triggers, they were elusive enough that years of monitoring did not reveal what they were.

We did eventually discover that our son's condition, specifically his outbursts and wild tantrums, would escalate with changes in the weather. My belief is that his heightened sensory stimulation was affected by changes in the barometric pressure, as perhaps this impacted his sensory system. It's just a guess. But we knew that when the weather changed drastically, so would our child. It became so obvious that we'd look at the local weather report to see if we were in for a "Big Norm Storm."

Over the years and as we worked with our child, we did learn to help him cope with some of these behavioral issues. We taught him how to redirect his anger, sadness, and other emotions so the duration of the episodes got shortened. Rather than being on the floor yelling, screaming, and kicking for three hours, we eventually got this down to about fifteen seconds. However, the outbursts continue to this day. He just has shorter episodes.

Many times throughout our son's life we discussed the impact of his specific condition. I hate to admit this, but we actually felt as if he'd be better off if he had a physical disability. Others might show him more compassion and understanding if they could physically see something wrong with him. But externally he looked fine, and in fact, he was very mobile. This added to the complexity of keeping him under control.

Finally, I'd like to describe our son's current mental state. He is sixteen years old now. However, mentally he's about a three-year-old in terms of his cognitive age. He can say his name and address but cannot spell or write it down. Most of his information is learned through his auditory senses (i.e., hearing). So he can listen to something and repeat it back but will shortly forget it. Our two hundred-pound three-year-old loves to watch TV and play with his cars. He pretends he's some of the characters on TV, which was the basis for the title of this book. I've often heard him saying, "I'm Superman" as he watches the TV shows. We'll say, "Come on, Superman, let's go to bed," and he'll react with that wide-eyed, lovable smile we've all fell in love with.

He's not the son I thought I'd have when our family began, but he's touched our hearts and changed our lives in more ways that any other child could have. Sometimes it's been difficult, more often than not. However, he's also had some very positive impacts on our family. I'll cover these blessings in the last chapter of this book, so we leave this subject on a high note.

Finally, I want to touch on the subject of family support. If you are a parent of an autistic child, make sure you accept any and all support your family offers. They may not always do what you want and may sometimes react inappropriately. But their intent is good, and your child more than likely needs all the help that can be provided. In our specific case, we were very private people and were initially not open to discussing our son's condition with our family. It wasn't their fault, just the result of us wanting to keep things to ourselves as we struggled inside to barely understand and deal with this horrible situation.

Years later it became obvious that we could not hide this issue from our family, as it impacted our ability to be with them. They were all very helpful and in their own ways, tried to help. However, as I mentioned, it's very difficult for anyone not living with this child to totally understand the complexity and significance of this illness. I believe many of our relatives just thought our son was slow, development wise. Although this was true, none of them could realize the violent emotional rage this child could unleash unexpectedly or the destruction he could cause. It just was not possible for anyone to imagine without actually experiencing it.

Even our doctors sometimes were unprepared for the things our son could dish out. I recall one time being at our son's doctor's office and he had taken something off her desk. She immediately came up to him and said, "Now please give that back," as she took it out of his hands. He immediately punched her in the stomach and laughed out loud and pushed everything off her desk. "Norman, stop. Tell the doctor you're sorry," I said as we ran over to him. "Doctor sorry," Norm said.

"You can make your next appointment with my secretary," the doctor replied. "Let's go for nine months," she added.

I guess she didn't want us back real soon. I wonder why? (Smile.)

This is about par for the course we've been on with few people really understanding the scope of our son's disability. However, it's vital that anyone caring for an autistic child realize that the child is very sick, not just bad. The behavioral outbursts, emotional flare ups, sensory uncontrollability, and mass destruction are all items beyond the child's level of control. Even when years are spent teaching specific behavioral and sensory techniques, in the end the condition still exists.

# CHAPTER 17

# PLANNING, PRIORITIZING, AND PURCHASING

We're now down to the home stretch. Hopefully by now, you know a little about what autism can do to your child, your life, and your family. You've got some items that should help you make some good decisions about which services would benefit your child, and the basics on how to quickly obtain these. You're also positioned to begin to restructure your financial world, so you can have the flexibility and freedom to make the decisions needed to best help your child.

This next chapter is an attempt to prioritize the real purchases you'll probably want to make so that you can do all this stuff to help your child. There's an endless list of things that can be purchased for an autistic or mentally retarded child. However, at the end of the day, there's really only a short list of items that you really need right now, aside from basic food, shelter, transportation, hygiene, and medical items. I'm going to make the assumption that you've already determined any special diet or medical supports needed for your child's condition.

I also will assume that you've taken care of any special transportation needs for your child, such as a car seat, safety harness, or special restraints. If you have not thought about it, some of the services, such as family-driven funds may help pay for special restraints, seat modifications, or other transportation-related adaptations needed for your vehicles if these are items needed to safely transport your disabled child. Discuss any such requests with your local MHMR case manager and then use the suggestions in the chapter on the power of print to go after them.

These items should be your first priority in terms of making sure your child is fed, clothed, medicated, safely transported, and has other items needed to maintain immediate health. I also will not discuss the subject of where to live. Everyone obviously needs a place to live, and given the destructive nature of our son's condition, we were blessed in having a home where he could live life out loud without bothering the neighbors. However, this subject is way beyond the scope of this book, and I'm just not comfortable going there. So I won't.

But what else do we need to buy for our special needs child, and in what order? This question is difficult to answer, so I'll simply provide some suggestions as to which items we found essential as we became the super-advocates for our child. Many of these items may seem simple or obvious depending on your career, experience, and other factors. However, I'm going to make no assumptions when it comes to clearly spelling these items out. If you're a young single parent trying to raise an autistic child, you may not be familiar with all these things. So I'm taking the time to list them out and explain why they are essential for your child's success.

The very first thing I'd suggest for a new parent to get for their autistic child and family is a good computer, with Internet connectivity. This item isn't for the child to use, it's for you. As I've documented in this book, there's a lot of research, reading, writing, and interaction needed to really become a good advocate for your child. As each day passes, there is also more information available regarding treatments for autism and the various support groups. You simply cannot perform all the actions needed to engage in these items without a good computer that has Internet connectivity. So get one. Trust me, if you're doing everything needed for your child to improve, it will be heavily used.

The second item you should consider buying is a good printer. The computer and printer do not need to be high-end devices. They simply need to be reliable and easy for you to use. In fact, you don't even need a color printer necessarily, just something to spew out the letters, responses, grievances, and appeals you'll be doing. Remember the section on the power of print. These tools are your sword and shield, so get them in place before you do battle.

If you are not familiar with how to use a computer, have someone close to you show you how to handle the basics. Or you can order something like the "video professor," which is a video showing you how to use different applications. When you're done, you need to be able to launch and search the Internet, create and print a Word document, and save files in an organized fashion. You should also install an electronic calendar or organizer so you can set schedule reminders and plan your child's appointments.

As previously mentioned, many service processes have set dates for responses or fixed appeal periods. Using an electronic scheduling tool (such as Microsoft Outlook or something equivalent) will make your life much simpler, more organized, and easier to plan. You'll have to schedule IEP meetings, doctors' appointments, and other critical engagements for your child. Doing this manually is a losing proposition and will eventually bite you.

So get these tools and learn how to use them. It'll be well worth the time spent. Remember I said I was going to cover the basics. So if you're already set with a computer, printer, and these applications, then you're ahead of the game. However, not everyone is already "connected," and having these items puts you in a far better position to be able to efficiently and effectively become a super-advocate for your child.

These next items are probably something you can get for free, but they are just as important as anything else. Make sure you have a current phone book and yellow page directory providing contact numbers for your local MHMR and the other service agencies in your area. You may have one, but it may be out of date. Get the most recent copy and put it somewhere so you can easily find it.

Next, you'll need some place to organize and store files. This should be something that's specifically targeted for your child's files and nothing else. A large two- or three-drawer file cabinet will suffice. Or you can use an old dresser or any place where you can put documents, organize paper files, and find them quickly. The point is that you will soon have many documents, write ups, plans, reports, and other material related to the assessment of your child's condition. Their IEP documentation alone will eventually fill a drawer of this cabinet. Make sure you set up the place for storing these items in advance of receiving them. Otherwise, you run the risk of losing or not finding these items when you need them most.

Keep all reports or assessments related to your child's condition *forever*. You never know when you may need to refer to them in order to fight for specific services, supports, or aides. Also remember, autistic children get into things and destroy them. So having a way to lock up the files isn't a bad idea. If the computer can be a laptop, which you can also lock up, maybe that's best. You need to decide the most effective way to do this, based on your finances, home environment, and other factors.

Next, make sure you have either an identification card with your child's name, address, and contact info—or at least have a recent photo on file of your child. There may be a way to get this done working with your child's local school district or teacher. You never know when you may have to give this to someone in the event that your child becomes lost. Update this information a minimum of annually or more frequently if your child's appearance drastically changes. And keep this information on file in a location where you can quickly and easily find it.

Other items to consider are the purchase of a medic alert bracelet or necklace providing any critical details as to allergies or other aspects of your child's medical condition. We decided not to go down this path, as the risk of our son biting the bracelet was more than the risk of not having the information available. However, we did put his name on the inside of his clothing and ensured that he could eventually say his name and address if asked. It wasn't a perfect solution, but it was a realistic one that worked best for our situation.

I suggest you not spend more than a thousand dollars on all of these items combined. You can easily get a very nice laptop or desktop computer with a printer included at Best Buy or other stores for well under $600. The balance of the funds should be used to set up Outlook, Word, and other applications, along with your Internet connectivity. You won't need a super high-speed Internet connection, but every little bit of speed helps with reducing the time you'll spend on these items. So plan, prioritize, and purchase, making these items the very first on your list.

The next item on your list should be a TV for your child to use with a VCR or DVD player. Over the years we found that our son learned a lot from listening to early childhood development tapes, such as the animal alphabet and other items like this. Make sure the TV isn't a high-end device, as they'll probably destroy it over time. Also, if you can mount the

TV out of your child's reach (such as behind some Plexiglas or high up on the wall using a mount), this would be best.

I'm not proposing that you just sit your child in a room, turn on the TV, and forget about them. However, don't assume that early educational TV programs designed for helping normal children develop won't help your child. There may be some significant benefits from being exposed to this material. And the ability to watch it over and over (and over and over) will allow your child to learn these items in his or her own special way over whatever time period is best. We also found that TV acted as a calming agent for our son after he became about twelve years old. We had to carefully monitor what programming was on, as he also could become excited if violent shows came on. However, if we turned on a cartoon channel, we could expect at least a few hours of quiet, peaceful tranquility.

The next item I'm proposing is a bit more costly, so consider this one for yourselves depending on your specific financial situation. We purchased the Hooked on Phonics program, and I sincerely recommend it for helping any child's development. But here's the fact—it didn't really help our son. It helped our other children. Remember I mentioned earlier in the book that the siblings of an autistic child often exhibit developmental delays as a result of being exposed to an autistic person during their early development. For our five other children, four of them had specific learning and language delays. The Hooked on Phonics program helped each of them catch up very quickly, and actually accelerated their learning abilities to the point where they are now honor roll students.

This was pretty cool to watch as our daughters went from being at the bottom of their class to the head of the class practically overnight. I really recommend this program for any families wishing to give their kids a head start in school. Remember, depending on the significance of your child's autism, it may or may not help with development, as the material may simply be beyond his or her level of comprehension. But if you have other children who could benefit from this kind of help, this is the program to use. Nothing comes close to its effectiveness, style, or results.

These next items are not related to your child's development. They are more focused on the family and maintaining your sanity in a very insane reality. Use these items as you see fit. Also remember that each of these items were things that we used daily, often several times a day. So consider purchasing a high-quality appliance, as the old saying is true, "You get what you pay for." You won't have time to fix, repair, or replace these items, as they'll only break when you need them the most. So if you can afford it, budget and plan for buying a quality item. You'll be glad you did in the long run.

Now we will focus on the security of your home, your child, and the things inside it. I'm including this due to an event we had when our son got out of our home while we were sleeping. My daughter came running into our room yelling, "The garage door is open and I can't find Norman!" *Oh no,* I thought. My wife and I ran downstairs to find exactly what my daughter had said. The garage door was open, the roll-up door was open, and Norman was no where to be seen. We immediately put on our clothes and got in the car, driving up and down the street. There was no sign of him.

We continued going up and down every street within about a one-mile radius around our home but didn't see him. Within about twenty minutes, we were terrified. Could he have wandered into the woods? Could he have been hit by a car? Or worse, could someone have taken him? Our worst fears mounted into terror as I picked up the phone and dialed 911. "Yes hello … uh … my autistic son is missing … my name … it's … we live at … What was he wearing? Heck, I don't know, probably a diaper … no … he's almost twelve … yes … in a diaper … He's totally unable to comprehend anything … we need help now!"

You can imagine the terror in my voice as I thought about all the bad things that could have happened. My wife began crying and everyone stared at me as I spoke to the operator. What could I have done to prevent this? Was it my fault? Would we ever get him back?

I'm very happy to say that as soon as I stopped stammering on the phone, the 911 operator said, "Officers have your son at this address." I asked, "Are you sure it's him?" and she said, "Oh yeah, we're pretty sure it's him." We immediately drove up the street, turned right, and there was our son sitting on someone's porch, pulling flowers out of their flower box. "I'm very sorry," I said as I approached the officers and the homeowners. "Is there anything we can do to make this up to you?" I asked the lady. "No," she said, "its fine." Her husband muttered something about, "Man, what's wrong with that kid," as they went into their house. I didn't care. I just wanted our son back safe and sound. And that day we were fortunate enough to get him back.

From that minute on, I immediately began to realize that we could not let our son be in an environment where he could leave unattended. The risk of being trapped was far less than the risk of him endangering himself by leaving during the night. So as a result, I installed dual-sided keyed deadbolts on all of the external doors to our home. I ensured our children had a clear understanding of how to exit in an emergency. However, on a day-by-day basis, these deadbolts remain locked. They've prevented our son from doing a repeat of this event, which I never want to go through again—ever.

So the point is to secure your child's environment to whatever degree is needed. Or put another way, invest $100 on some good locks strategically placed to keep your child safe. You may want to secure your child's bedroom door or your front and side house doors. You may want to lock windows so there's no risk of falling or jumping out of a second-story window. Your specific needs will vary from ours, but the end point is the same—keep your child within your control at all times.

Other people may not understand what this is about and may actually say you're being cruel when they see locks on the outside of your child's bedroom door. None of them can even imagine the difficulty, anguish, or pain that parents of these kinds of kids go through as they struggle to keep their kids safe. I do not recommend that you lock any child into an environment without proper monitoring. So whether it's installing a video camera, a peep window, or other mechanisms, make sure you monitor your child at all times. Baby monitoring systems are a good way to make this happen. But work within your own budget and do what makes sense for you and your family.

Door locks may also be appropriate for your bedroom and other areas of the home where valuables are kept. One thing we found in our battle against autism is that it brought many new strangers into our lives, and often into our house. I won't say whether anything was taken from our home, but let's just say people will be people. Restricting access is an important part of maintaining control in your life, especially when strangers are involved in your home. So lock up places that you don't want just anyone to wander into.

As we expanded our understanding of our son's unique needs, we eventually fenced in our entire backyard. We felt that there was just too much risk of him wandering off, falling in a neighbor's pool, or going after one of the dogs in the neighborhood. This was a much larger expense, and we were fortunate enough to have family-driven funds help pay a portion of the cost. Remember to consider using the services previously mentioned to help augment the cost of some of these items. It might not pay for all of them or cover the entire cost, but every little bit helps especially if you're a one-income family.

Finally I secured our garage, basement, and any area where I had tools. I probably should have done this for any child in our home; however, it became quickly obvious that our son's condition would make these areas a high risk for injuring himself. I secured the door to the garage with a keyed deadbolt, locked up all the sharp tools, and made sure we stored items appropriately. This didn't cost a lot, but the ounce of prevention was well worth it. You may also want to double check the chemicals and other cleaning agents in your home. Normally parents are asked to put these up high, to prevent small children from getting into them. However, since autistic children are very mobile and grow large in size, you may find that it's better to put any chemicals or cleaning substances behind locked doors to prevent any chance of someone swallowing them. Do not depend on these being located up high, as they could be easily reached by your child when you're not looking.

One good thing to remember is, "No metals, no magnets, no sharps, and no solutions." If you keep these kinds of objects out of your child's reach, you will prevent many of these potentially serious injuries from ever occurring. Plastic items can also cause damage, so don't think you can let your guard down. However, in most cases this will be far less of a risk than the damage that could occur when ingesting metals, magnets, sharp objects, or chemical cleaning solutions.

This next item was purchased for my wife, and it was one of the major keys to help us stay successfully married during this experience. No, it wasn't a holiday in the Caribbean. It was a good, commercial-sized rug cleaner to address the big, commercial-sized messes our son made each day.

As you'll recall, our son had an issue with keeping the contents of his diaper in his diaper. I won't get into details on this subject, as it stinks.

However, normal vacuums and carpet cleaners just could not handle these large catastrophes. We purchased several dozen makes and models of carpet cleaning devices and finally bought one that did what the manufacturer claimed. If you're faced with a similar set of circumstances, go out and buy the wide-sized Rug Doctor carpet cleaning system. It's not cheap (about $600 when we got it years ago), but it's worth every penny. Also, if you can afford it, get all the upholstery attachments that go with it. These attachments can be used to quickly clean the walls and ceilings, if needed.

You can try other cheaper devices if you want, but I'm fairly sure that eventually you'll come to the conclusions we did. This is the only device we've found that is available for residential use that provides the cleaning power needed for these kinds of disasters. This device greatly improved our ability to keep our home clean, resolve those "special presents" our son would create for us, and keep our sanity through all the madness.

If you want to purchase the cleaning agents through the Rug Doctor retailer, that's fine. However, we found these to be a bit too expensive given the frequency we had to clean things up. Instead, we purchased some of the oxy-type cleaning agents from our local dollar store and added a small amount to some warm water, along with some Resolve carpet cleaning mix. The solution did a great job of cleaning up the mess, getting rid of the smell, and keeping the color of our carpets from fading. I highly recommend that anyone considering use of this method for cleaning their own carpets, upholstery, or curtains perform a test on a small hidden area before doing this on a large-scale area. The color fastness or fading of your carpets may not be the same as ours, and each person should test their specific home environment before proceeding. Otherwise you may seriously damage the items in your home. Just use caution and good common sense before you go out and clean your world. However, if your experience is like ours, these items will be a gift from heaven.

There's one other thing I'd like you to know, and it's regarding the best way for retrieving items that are flushed down the toilet. Our son would continually flush items down the toilet, many of which would become stuck or lodged in place. At first, I pulled the toilet off its mount to get these items out. But as you can probably imagine, this quickly became more hassle than it is worth. I tried using tools to go in and get the items, but nothing worked, as the toilet has bends and curves, making a straight retrieval impossible. What finally worked was using the hose from a Wet-Vac (or your Rug Doctor) to suck the water out of the toilet first, then snake the hose into the toilet to grab the item. We actually had a Wet-Vac with a 1.5-inch hose that worked very well. This became an essential part of our daily routine as our son "plugged up" the toilet each day. Rather than get mad, I'd just get the Wet-Vac, put on my gloves, suck it out, and get on with life. Worked like a champ!

Okay, we're down to the last two items I'm recommending. Are you out of money yet? If so, that's okay. Just put together your prioritized list of what you think works best for your family, and plan for these expenses as the funds become available. It's not as if you'll fail immediately if you don't have all these items in your home tomorrow morning. We just found that of all the things we bought over the years, these are the things that made a huge difference, regardless of the cost. So hopefully some of these items will also be a benefit to you and your family.

Next we found that keeping our son clothed, showered, and groomed was a bit more challenging that any person could endure. I've already discussed the clothing aspect of his condition and shared ways to deal with his continual shredding behaviors. Also make sure you have a good, reliable washer and dryer to perform the cleaning needed for your special child. There will be monumental-sized messes each day. Although any washer or dryer will initially do, I highly suggest you purchase a good reliable washer and dryer set when the timing is right, when you can afford it. You will use it for your child and your family, and it will be money well spent.

Showers were another story, as he would not get into any shower—ever. So we had to install a shower head with a long hose, so we could shower him in the bathroom open area. We used a plastic bin from Wal-Mart on the floor to collect the water. We would shower him, dump the water, and clean up any spillage each morning. It's not a perfect solution, but it allows us to clean him easily and not fight the mother of all battles each day.

Finally, let's discuss hair cuts. Oh boy, hold onto your hat, as here we go! We initially took our son to a barber who said he had worked with all kinds of autistic kids. We thought everything would be okay—but of course, we should have known better. After about three hours of our son running around the store yelling at the top of his lungs, the barber finally got him to sit on the floor and came up to him to begin gently cutting his hair. Our son yelled as each strand of hair was cut, as if the barber was cutting the nerve endings in his head. Could our son actually feel it? I didn't know. However, we got about a quarter of one side of his head cut and then were asked to pay the $20 for the haircut. The barber could not get this done—and we were left without a solution.

So after shopping around a bit and thinking about it, we purchased a Flowbee hair-cutting system off of the Internet. This is a device you hook to your vacuum and the suction pulls the hair into a scissor mechanism that cuts it. My wife and I both had to physically hold my son down, but we got his hair cut. It was actually much safer than going near him with scissors or any sharp, unprotected blades. We've continued to use this method to cut his hair for years. I'm fairly convinced that we've not only kept him safe and well groomed, but we also probably saved a few dollars over the long haul. The Flowbee cost about $80 and can be easily ordered online via the Internet.

# CHAPTER 18

# EXPECT THE UNEXPECTED
# AS IT CAN BE WONDERFUL!

So here we are. You've made it to the final chapter! By now you should have at least some idea of what my wife and I went through and some understanding of the items we felt really helped us become the best advocates we could for our special Superman. I think it's time to describe some of the good things we experienced as we fought the battle of our lives. "Good things?" you may ask. How the heck can anyone experience good things when going through this kind of hell?

I'll try to tackle this subject a bit more in my second book, *Ten-inch Nails*. But for now, let's just say we're alive and thriving as a family. Of course, our lives are very different from those around us. And our oldest son will never become the doctor or rocket scientist I had hoped for when he was born. These are realities we simply have to live with.

However, if the truth be known, our son has impacted all of our lives more than any normal son could ever have done, in many very positive ways. As an example, my wife and I have become a true team working for the betterment of our son and family. We always loved each other before he was born. However, over the years of struggle, we learned to appreciate each other in ways that each of us previously could not have imagined.

We learned to work as a team, truly respecting each other for our diversity, differences, and challenges. She learned to respect my engagement, negotiation, and process skills. I learned to appreciate her dedication, hard work, stable temperament, and balance in the midst of adversity. I come to her for her opinion now, on the most complex and demanding items that occur in my life. This kind of communication and interaction never occurred before my son was born. It was a direct result of us working together as one team, for our son's success.

We also raised a beautiful family together. After our son was born, we had our first daughter about two years later. We had not quite figured out how sick our son was. Fortunately, when we had her, she was fine. Otherwise, we might have been paralyzed with fear about having more kids with autism. But as things turned out, she was already born, she was fine, and so we figured what the heck—let's have some more. And we did. We had four more children altogether, for a total of six children. It's a blast, and every day is a party!

All of our children have worked hard in supporting our oldest son, and each of them has a clear and unique understanding of what's important in life. I believe in our specific case, having more children actually helped with our ability to deal with the mental and spiritual anguish that came with these events. Had all our hopes and dreams been tied up into our only son, then I think we would have been devastated by his disability. Initially I was concerned that having more children would dilute our focus to address his special needs. But this turned out to be the exact opposite of what really occurred. Our other children stepped right up and tried to help in any manner they could. As they got older, each took on whatever role was needed to help supervise and guide our son. Finally, as a group they developed into some of the most wonderful, mature, and responsible folks I've ever met.

They're very understanding about other children with special needs and don't judge people by their external appearances or disabilities. They've also worked hard to help, love, and challenge each other. I'm very proud of them. Despite all the negative issues our oldest son experienced, it's obvious that his disabilities brought us all closer together and forced us to become a real family. I also want to take a moment and personally thank all of my children for their support as they've helped us raise our son. Lea, Jennifer, Jessica, Danielle, and Howard Jr. have all been wonderful as we went for this long roller coaster ride in the fog. What about my wife? Well let's just say I wouldn't be here writing this book if it wasn't for her. She's the magic that lights up my world!

These aren't trivial successes, as I don't see many families having the closeness, love, and nurturing relationships we share at home. I actually want to come home each night, even though on several nights it's likely I'll have to get the Wet-Vac and Rug Doctor out. (Smile.) Even with those challenges, our son's positive impact on our lives has caused our family to blossom from dirt into a wonderful garden. Each of our kids has flourished, and our relationships have grown as a result of this experience.

Remember that the things you get help improve how you live. But the things you give help you improve your life! Raising a child with significant autism either makes or breaks you as a person and as a family. If you step up to the challenge, you can almost guarantee that you'll be a tight-knit group of folks who live and love together. There's no choice but to commit to a life of service in support of your child, especially if you love your children as much as we love ours. These events forced us to spend time as a family and learn to appreciate life's little rewards.

The continuous financial and supervisory requirements of our son's condition forced us to seriously consider whether we could be a one or two-income family. Finally, after we realized that my wife had to stay home to support him, we had to deal with some serious financial realities. We got out of debt early, and we stayed out of debt. For over sixteen years, we've never fought about money—ever. This was something I never would have imagined as a benefit to raising a child who's this sick. However, rather than split us up, destroy our marriage, and take our focus off our other children, this experience has brought us closer together in a manner I could never have expected. Not a bad trade, eh?

Finally, if I can offer one word of advice to those who are faced with a similar challenge, it would be to never give up and don't get discouraged. It was years before I realized that the best we could do was simply the best we could do. We could not be perfect, as our son was Superman. However, we were not. There were many very bad days and very long nights.

But fortunately, there were also some very good ones. We didn't forget to enjoy the ride, and I encourage each of you to do the same. Be very proud of the work you're doing as the super-advocate for your child. Realize that raising any child, especially one with significant disabilities, is a very

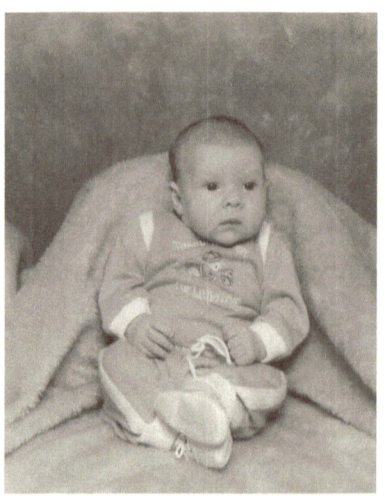
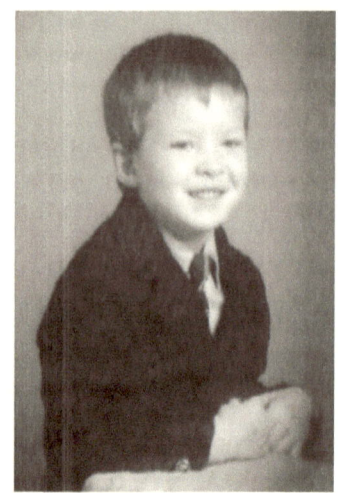

complex, demanding, and difficult task. You deserve a medal just for being involved and staying by their side. Don't depend on the feedback from others to feel good about your child, your progress, or your results. Few, if any people on the planet have any clue as to what you're up against.

Many years ago I heard someone say that God has "special angels" to watch over special needs children. I'm not sure if that's true, but one thing is for certain. God has made special people to watch over special needs children, and you're one of them! Otherwise, you wouldn't be spending your time reading this book.

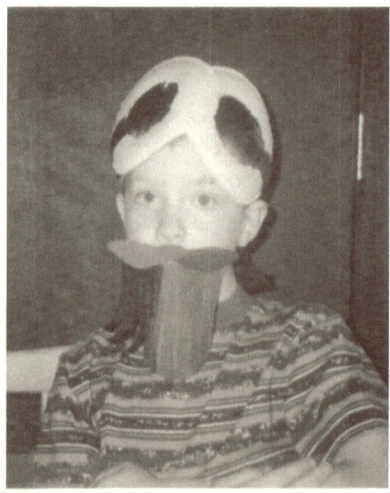
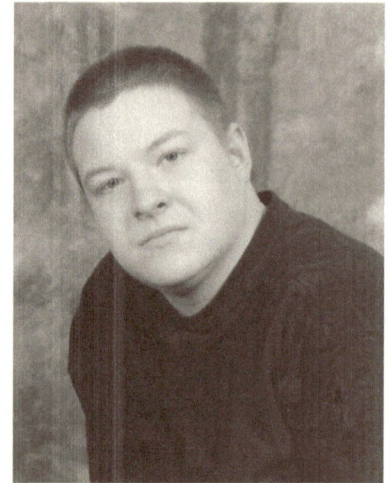

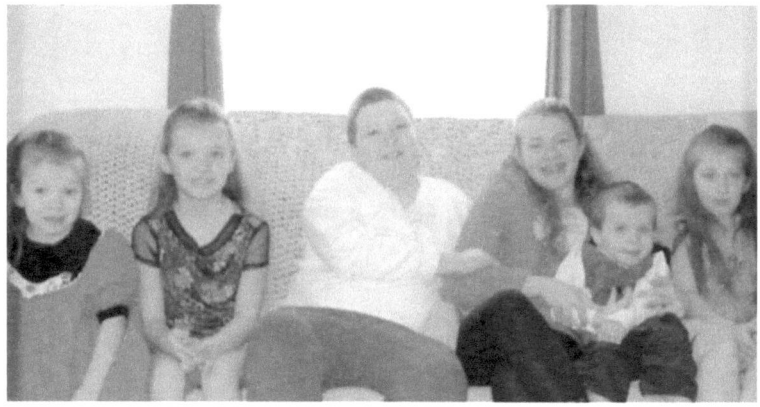

So be proud as you win those little victories. Take the time to celebrate successes with your family. Allow yourself to rest, recharge, and re-engage to fight the good fight. And remember, when we all get to heaven, your little super-special angel and your family will be there with open arms to hug, thank, and love you for all you did!

*May god bless you, give you the strength, wisdom, and courage to do your very best, and bring your family nothing but happiness—forever!*

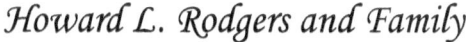

*Howard L. Rodgers and Family*

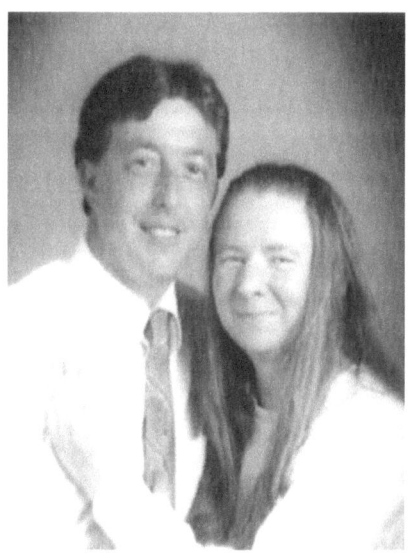

www.ingramcontent.com/pod-product-compliance
Lightning Source LLC
Chambersburg PA
CBHW030342290526
45785CB00004B/1571